JUST DIAGNOSED

JUST DIAGNOSED

A SURVIVOR'S GUIDE *to* NAVIGATING CANCER

JENNIFER OMHOLT

Foreword by Debu Tripathy, MD
The University of Texas MD Anderson Cancer Center

SWP
SHE WRITES PRESS

Published in 2026 by
She Writes Press, an imprint of The Stable Book Group

32 Court Street, Suite 2109
Brooklyn, NY 11201
https://shewritespress.com
The Library of Congress Control Number is available upon request.
ISBN: 979-8-89636-202-9
eISBN: 979-8-89636-203-6

Interior Designer: Tabitha Lahr

Printed in the United States

Medical Disclaimer

This book is for informational purposes only and is not intended as a substitute for professional medical advice, diagnosis, or treatment. The content reflects the author's personal experiences, research, and insights, but should not be interpreted as medical guidance.

Readers should always seek the advice of a qualified healthcare professional regarding any medical concerns or treatment decisions. Never disregard professional medical advice or delay seeking it based on information presented in this book.

The author and publisher disclaim any responsibility for adverse effects resulting from the use of information contained in this book. Each person's medical situation is unique, and treatment decisions should always be made in consultation with a licensed healthcare provider.

Errors and Omissions Disclaimer

Every effort has been made to ensure the accuracy and completeness of the information presented in this book. However, medical knowledge is constantly evolving, and errors or omissions may occur. Neither the author nor the publisher assumes responsibility for any inaccuracies, errors, or omissions, or for any outcomes resulting from the use of this book.

The author and publisher expressly disclaim liability for any adverse effects, consequences, or damages resulting from the use or misuse of the information contained herein.

For everyone whose life has been touched by cancer—
patients, caregivers, and those who love them.

May this book be a steady companion in
times of uncertainty and a source of strength
and hope along the way.

Contents

Foreword

A diagnosis of cancer is an unexpected and unfathomable turn in one's life. It activates a myriad of emotions and visceral reactions like fear, anger, and disbelief. At the same time, in recent years, tremendous progress has been made in the management of cancer that has made this disease more curable than ever before. And even when a cure is not possible, advances in treatment continue to improve survival and quality of life at an increasingly rapid pace.

Discovering you have cancer can unleash a flood of questions and an urgent need for guidance. Having access to information that is easy to understand and that can be tailored to your own situation can be highly valuable.

Jennifer Omholt's *Just Diagnosed* is a refreshing and rich resource for patients, as well as their families, friends, and caregivers. Drawing from her insights and experiences as a cancer survivor and her network of professional resources, she has created a comprehensive and well-organized guidebook from which readers can benefit by perusing the most appropriate chapter, given their current needs.

The preface to *Just Diagnosed* opens with a quote that sets the emotional tone for the book: "*You can't stop the waves, but you can learn to surf.*" Its author, Jon Kabat-Zinn—a professor, biologist, and founder of the Stress Reduction Clinic and the Center for Mindfulness in Medicine—revolutionized the field of mindfulness-based stress reduction (MBSR). A thread that runs throughout the book—especially in the opening chapter—is the importance of anchoring yourself in the present moment. Calmly noticing your thoughts, feelings, and physical sensations is at the heart of MBSR, a meditative discipline that has been formally studied in the context of cancer and shown to offer both emotional and physical benefits. The simple yet elegant practice of breathwork can be beneficial at this and other junctures of the cancer journey, as detailed early in this book.

Alongside practices that foster grounding and reflection, *Just Diagnosed* offers essential practical information to support early decision-making. The first days after diagnosis often involve a steep learning curve. Patients are introduced to complex medical terms, diagnostic tests, treatment options, and staging systems that determine prognosis. They may feel overwhelmed as they try to understand the biology of their cancer, the expected side effects of treatment, and the big-picture implications for their future.

Patients are often surprised by how many decisions need to be made shortly after diagnosis, including choosing (or being assigned or referred to) the members of their treatment team, including oncologists and other medical specialists, nurses, pharmacists, genetic counselors, and potentially other disciplines. While patients may not be able to make all these choices for themselves, valuable tips are provided in this section on how to make the best connections.

The first part of *Just Diagnosed* reviews this difficult stage of diagnosis and the several steps that may be involved in treatment planning—sometimes requiring additional tissue and blood tests, as well as imaging studies. Throughout this section, Jennifer emphasizes the importance of involving trusted loved ones in weighing options and making decisions. She reminds readers that they—and their inner circle—are not passive participants but active partners in care. Then there is the "larger community"—online resources that have blossomed over the last decade or two and made cancer information not only more accessible and user-friendly but also transactional and service-oriented. These are very well described in Chapter 2, along with ways to leverage social media for updates and services that are tailored to newly diagnosed cancer patients.

As Jennifer points out with her own story, the principle of self-advocacy is not only centering but also empowering. It reminds us that speaking up isn't a challenge to authority—it's a commitment to one's own well-being. Trusting one's instincts, even when they run counter to expert advice, can make the difference between a good outcome and a regrettable one. Sometimes this means seeking a second opinion—especially when the tradeoffs between treatments, side effects, and outcomes feel uncertain. Most of us never expect to be faced with such decisions, but Part Two of this book equips readers to make informed choices with clarity and confidence.

Patients today have access to detailed, evidence-based treatment guidelines from professional organizations. These guidelines consider tumor type, stage, biochemical, genetic and genomic features, and personal factors. They also highlight supportive care measures: how to manage side effects, preserve fertility, seek psychosocial support, and integrate complementary therapies such as meditation, yoga, or guided imagery—when appropriate and when supported by data.

The pace of progress in cancer treatment is accelerating. Promising new therapies are frequently approved, and others may be available through clinical trials. Yet accessing trials requires careful planning, specific eligibility criteria, and sometimes travel to specialty centers. Jennifer explains this complex process with lucidity in Chapter 11 and provides guidance on how to search for appropriate studies. She underscores the importance of partnering with your oncologist to navigate the eligibility process and explore clinical trial options that align with your treatment goals.

Staying organized about your health is always important—but it becomes challenging when you're facing cancer or other medical issues. Organizational strategies are therefore tantamount and not easily implemented without the systematic approach that is provided in Part Three for communicating with employers, insurers, pharmacies, and medical billing offices. While some of this information may exist online or through individual employers, this section empowers patients to navigate bureaucracy with greater ease.

Part Four explores practical strategies and emerging science that help patients build emotional and physical resilience—a process that infuses survival with function and grace. Resilience can be intrinsic or developed over time through nutritional and behavioral adaptations that enhance quality of life. Although research in this area is still evolving, this section explains the science behind these strategies and offers guidance on how to adapt them to your lifestyle and resources.

The chapter on emotional support illustrates how meaningful connection can be just as vital to healing as medical treatment. With vulnerability and insight, Jennifer shares how isolation gave way to profound relief through support groups and peer relationships—bonds that not only eased her loneliness but also influenced her care in lasting ways. She guides readers through the many types of support available, from group settings to one-on-one mentorship, and presents evidence that these connections can enhance both quality of life and survival. Blending personal experience with practical tools and trusted resources, she reassures newly diagnosed patients that they don't have to face cancer alone—and affirms that reaching out for support is a courageous step toward healing.

One of the great strengths of *Just Diagnosed* is its clear, compelling presentation of mind-body techniques that are becoming increasingly accessible to patients. Jennifer not only demystifies these practices but also grounds them in evidence, reflecting the growing body of research that supports their use. Organizations like the Society for Integrative Oncology have developed rigorous, evidence-based guidelines for complementary therapies that clinical trials have shown to have meaningful benefits for cancer patients.

Empowering patients with knowledge and confidence is a pillar of good cancer care. *Just Diagnosed* is a timely and thoughtful contribution to the resources available to patients and the broader cancer community.

Debu Tripathy, MD
Professor of Medicine and Former Chair
Department of Breast Medical Oncology
The University of Texas MD Anderson Cancer Center

Preface

"You can't stop the waves, but you can learn to surf."
—JON KABAT-ZINN, *Wherever You Go, There You Are*

Few experiences are as terrifying as a cancer diagnosis. Shockingly, it is in this fragile state of mind that you're expected to make critical treatment decisions. As a seasoned journalist, newly diagnosed with stage 3 breast cancer, I turned to research. But as someone reeling from the trauma, I found the information overwhelming and nearly impossible to process. Determined to find a practical guide to help me navigate the confusion, I soon realized that what I needed didn't exist—so I set out to create it, not just for myself, but for others facing the same daunting journey.

If you, too, feel like you don't know which end is up, know this: *You are not a statistic.*

Every day, people with cancer defy the odds. Studies address average treatment outcomes, but survival rates vary widely by cancer type, age, health, lifestyle, and ethnicity. No patient wants to be reduced to a percentage or told they only have so many months to live. The truth is—no one really knows.

Just Diagnosed transforms fear into actionable steps designed to bolster your confidence. It speaks to those poignant moments when you and your loved ones are desperate for practical information on how to proceed. As a grateful cancer survivor of more than twenty years, I feel compelled to share what I did to regain control after receiving a life-threatening diagnosis. My journey back to health was grounded in my firm belief: The more actively patients participate in their care, the greater their chances of healing—and surviving.

You don't need to implement every strategy presented here. In fact, it's essential to trust your intuition and choose the approaches that resonate with you. Healing is deeply personal, and what works for one person may not work for another. Give yourself the freedom to adjust along the way, trusting that your needs will likely evolve.

It is an honor to walk beside you as you navigate the uncertainty of these early days.

Author's Note

How to Use This Book in the Critical Early Days

This book was created to meet you exactly where you are, no matter how you choose to use it. Some readers will read it from cover to cover, while others will scan the table of contents and jump to whatever feels most pressing. Either approach works. What matters is that you find the guidance you need, when you need it.

In the days right after a diagnosis, you're expected to make critical medical decisions while emotionally overwhelmed and still trying to get your bearings. Yet certain early choices can significantly affect your treatment and long-term outcome. This section highlights a few of the most time-sensitive considerations to help you get oriented—fast.

- **Where to start.** A key consideration is whether your care would be best managed by a coordinated medical team rather than a single provider. If you're newly diagnosed with early-stage cancer, such as breast cancer, you may need to see both a surgical and a medical oncologist. It's ideal to begin at a center where these teams already collaborate and have shared access to your imaging and test results. For more complex diagnoses, such as brain metastases, inflammatory breast cancer, or pregnancy-associated cancer, you may want to begin care at a larger community hospital or academic medical center. These are just a few examples. Your first priority is to begin care in a setting equipped to meet your full range of needs.

- **Confirming your diagnosis.** Ensure your diagnosis has been reviewed by someone outside of your original care team and that you fully understand the nature of your cancer. Chapter 10: *Seek Second Opinions* walks you through how to do this.

- **Metastatic or advanced cancer.** Molecular testing, also called genomic sequencing, can play a critical role in determining the most effective treatment for metastatic or advanced cancer. As a key component of precision medicine, it allows doctors to tailor therapies based on the unique genetic profile of your tumor rather than relying on a one-size-fits-all approach. Chapter 5: Discover Your Treatment Options explores this, along with other important factors that can influence your treatment plan. Keep in mind that access to precision medicine can vary significantly depending on your cancer type, where you live, and the healthcare resources available to you.

- **Fertility preservation.** If you're of childbearing age and may want to have children in the future, bring this up as soon as possible—before treatment begins. Chapter 5: Discover Your Treatment Options outlines fertility preservation choices and helps you make informed decisions early.

- **Surgical planning.** Don't rush into surgery without understanding your options. Minimally invasive approaches and preoperative systemic therapy may help reduce the extent of surgery needed. Chapter 9: Make the Most of Medical Appointments walks you through seeking a multidisciplinary evaluation and preparing for conversations with your surgeon and oncology team.

- **Advance care planning.** This may feel premature, but hospitals now routinely ask about decision-making preferences, power of attorney, and resuscitation status at the first visit. This list isn't exhaustive. Your priorities may vary based on your diagnosis, age, values, and personal circumstances.

A quick note about web links: This book contains numerous URLs to trusted resources. If you find that a link no longer works, simply search the organization's name directly to access the most current information.

I encourage you to use the table of contents as a road map. If you're not sure where to begin, start with Chapter 1: Take a Deep Breath. It offers grounding practices that can help you steady yourself—and begin to move forward.

With compassion and strength,
Jennifer Omholt

PART ONE

COMING TO TERMS WITH YOUR DIAGNOSIS

Chapter 1

Take a Deep Breath

"Regulate the breath, and thereby control the mind."
—SVĀTMĀRĀMA, *Hatha Yoga Pradipika*

When you first hear the words "You have cancer," everything changes in an instant. There's a sudden rupture in reality. The life you knew is replaced with one marked by fear and the dreaded unknown.

My first suspicion of cancer struck me while sitting in my mother's living room in Albuquerque, helping plan my stepfather's memorial service. As I absentmindedly touched my breast, my fingers discovered a lump the size of a golf ball. My OB-GYN had been trying to reach me for days but, caught up in the chaos of grief and planning, I hadn't returned his calls. Looking back, I realize I was in denial. It wasn't until I was driving home from the airport that I finally called him back.

His voice was urgent. "We need to talk about your mammogram," he said firmly. I had put off getting one while nursing because I knew it would be painful and I was afraid of the results. When I gave birth at forty-two, I knew that my age put me at greater risk of breast cancer.

My doctor then asked if I had an infection in my upper arm, explaining that the radiologist had noticed swollen lymph nodes. When I told him I wasn't aware of any infection, he urged me to schedule a "mag view" immediately. He explained that a mag view was a specialized mammogram for detailed imaging. I scheduled it as soon as I got home. Soon after, I sat in the office of a breast surgeon, anxiously awaiting the results.

"The mass looks like a polar bear in a snowstorm," she said. "There's less than a 4 percent chance this is cancer."

My surgeon's confident prediction stood in stark contrast to the reality I would soon face.

"Then let's get rid of it!" I said, unaware of the risks of cutting into a potentially cancerous mass. I didn't realize that cutting into a tumor can dislodge cancer cells, potentially spreading them to the bloodstream or surrounding tissues. Learning this later—after the fact—left me questioning the choices I made and the guidance I received during those critical early moments.

Two weeks later, my surgeon performed the lumpectomy. When I woke up in the post-op room, she stood beside me, her expression guarded.

"I'm sorry, Jen. We couldn't get clean margins," she said apologetically.

I would eventually learn that if a cancerous tumor is not fully removed with "clean margins"—a rim of healthy tissue surrounding the tumor—there is a greater chance that cancer will recur at the site.

"Clean margins?" I repeated, disbelief flooding my voice.

She remained calm, almost clinical. "We'll know more when the pathology report comes back."

Later, my oncologist explained that because the cancer had not been fully removed, starting chemotherapy as soon as possible was critical. Unfortunately, chemotherapy suppresses the immune system and impairs the body's ability to heal wounds, meaning we had to wait for my surgical wound to heal first. This anxiety-inducing delay ultimately gave what turned out to be a very aggressive cancer more time to progress.

As I lay on the cold, sterile gurney, fear surged through me. Why had she cut into my breast, knowing the lump might be cancerous? Why hadn't she waited for the results of the sentinel lymph node biopsy I'd instinctively scheduled? I hadn't understood enough to insist that she wait for the results—and now, it was too late.

Looking back, I wondered, "Why hadn't I sought a second opinion? Could that one choice have impacted my odds of surviving this deadly disease?"

When my surgeon called with my pathology results, I was having lunch at a local haunt with my husband and my father, visiting from Philadelphia.

As she spoke, "stage 3 breast cancer" kept echoing in my head.

I was paralyzed by shock and an overwhelming sense of betrayal.

By my doctor.

By my own body.

The thought of my sixteen-month-old son growing up without me unleashed a torrent of tears.

A wave of nausea and disbelief sent me staggering to the nearest bathroom—a surreal moment seared into my memory.

Desperate to shake off this nightmare, I splashed cold water on my face. As the ground seemed to shift beneath me, I drew in several deep breaths, clinging to any grounding I could find as my world began to unravel. In that moment, focusing on my breath became an unexpected lifeline, anchoring me through the chaos.

That brief, grounding moment led me to explore the profound benefits of deep breathing, a practice central to many healing traditions. Modern research confirms its benefits, from reducing stress to improving immune function and lowering blood pressure.[1]

How Breath Supports Your Healing

Deep breathing is a simple yet powerful way to calm the nervous system, enhance focus, and ease stress-related symptoms. Practicing deep breathing regularly—at home, while waiting at appointments, or while receiving treatment—can be a valuable tool for alleviating the physical and emotional burden of anxiety, stress, and depression.

According to James Nestor, a reporter for *The Wall Street Journal* and author of *The New York Times* bestseller *Breath: The New Science of a Lost Art*, the first step in healthy breathing is extending your breaths to make them deeper and longer. Research indicates that just a few minutes of inhaling and exhaling at a slower pace can decrease blood pressure.[2] The second step in healthy breathing is breathing through your nose. Nasal breathing improves oxygen absorption by filtering, warming, and humidifying the air before it reaches the lungs.

Getting Started: Simple Breathing Techniques

We'll start with diaphragmatic breathing to help you take deeper, fuller breaths. Then we'll try triangular breathing, a simple tool to help you feel calm and centered, wherever you may be.

Both techniques will help you:

- Reduce anxiety and stress
- Enhance focus and clarity
- Improve oxygenation
- Lower blood pressure
- Regulate emotions
- Increase resilience to physical discomfort

▶ Diaphragmatic Breathing

Diaphragmatic breathing taps into the calming power of slow, intentional breaths. As you inhale and exhale, imagine a wave of soothing energy rising from your feet, moving gently up through your legs and torso, and flowing out through the top of your head. Each breath you take is a quiet but meaningful step toward healing.

STEP 1: Find a comfortable position. You can lie down with your knees bent or sit in a chair with your feet flat on the floor. Choose whichever feels best.

STEP 2: Place one hand on your chest and the other on your belly. This helps you notice how your breath is moving through your body.

STEP 3: Slowly breathe in through your nose. Let your belly rise under your hand as the air flows in. Try to keep your chest as still as possible.

STEP 4: Exhale gently through pursed lips. You might imagine softly blowing out a candle. As you breathe out, feel your belly soften and fall. Imagine breathing out all the tension in your body.

STEP 5: Continue for five to ten minutes, paying attention to the steady rhythm of your breath. It's OK if your mind wanders. That's natural. Just gently bring your attention back to your breath.

▶ Triangular Breathing

If you only have a minute or two, triangular breathing is a quick and effective way to steady your mind and body. Practice this simple technique wherever you go, and calm will become your constant companion.

STEP 1: Inhale deeply through your nose to a slow count of four.

STEP 2: Hold your breath for another count of four.

STEP 3: Exhale gently for a count of four.

STEP 4: Repeat four times.

With each breath, you're not just calming your mind, you're reclaiming control and taking a powerful step toward healing.

If you'd like to explore additional mind-body and meditative practices like the ones that helped me over the course of my journey, you'll find them in Part Five: Boost Your Mind, Body, and Spirit. These practices include:

- Meditation
- Guided imagery
- Somatic yoga
- Jin Shin Jyutsu
- Qigong
- Feldenkrais
- Reiki
- Healing affirmations

Chapter 2

Deliver the News to Friends and Family

"Friendship improves happiness and abates misery, by the doubling of our joy and the dividing of our grief."
—CICERO, *De Amicitia*

In the first few weeks after my diagnosis, I spent far too much time on the phone, repeating the painful news to family and friends. With every conversation, I relived the fear, confusion, and heartbreak. I often found myself in the absurd position of consoling the very people I'd called.

This zapped what little energy I had.

After a cancer diagnosis, your energy becomes one of your most precious resources—and you'll need to protect it fiercely. Sharing the news can be exhausting. Each conversation forces you to revisit the pain and uncertainty of your situation. To preserve your strength for what truly matters—your healing—keep your communication brief, intentional, and focused.

Rather than spreading yourself thin, centralize your updates. Lean on the people who've offered to help by asking them to take on this outreach. This isn't just about managing logistics, it's about creating space for peace, conserving your energy, and nurturing your emotional reserves for what lies ahead.

To protect your fragile state of mind and preserve your strength, I recommend that you ask someone you trust to help you draft a concise email about your diagnosis and initial treatments. Your outreach is an ideal opportunity to ask for medical referrals and resources.

Let others know that, until you send out a "green light" message, you would prefer not to receive calls. Instead, encourage them to reach out through email, text, or a card if they want to offer support. Once you feel ready to speak to friends and family, keep your phone time to a minimum. You need to reserve your energy for the next phase of your journey.

Centralized Communication Resources

Managing communication can reduce stress and help preserve your emotional energy during treatment. Consider offsetting the burden of one-to-one communication with private online forums that reach your entire community of family and friends.

Here are a few platforms that can help streamline updates and keep your community informed:

- **CaringBridge.org**
  CaringBridge lets you create a personal, secure website to share updates, your health status, and journal entries. With your own private community, you can share updates, and friends and family can leave messages of support and encouragement. CaringBridge also offers tools that help manage the logistical aspects of caregiving, such as visiting schedules, meal deliveries, and help with errands.

- **MyLifeLine.org**
  MyLifeLine is a part of Gilda's Club Cancer Support Community. Its goal is to reduce stress, anxiety, and isolation for newly diagnosed cancer patients by helping them connect with a supportive community. Like CaringBridge, it provides you with private community websites to keep family and friends updated and lets you control who can view your updates and personal stories.

  MyLifeLine is particularly valuable for its ability to adapt to the unique needs of cancer patients. For instance, the site offers access to a wider community of cancer patients and survivors, which can be crucial for emotional support and practical advice. The site also provides resources about cancer treatments, side effects, and patient support programs.

- **Lotsa Helping Hands**
  A community-based platform that coordinates meal deliveries, rides, and companionship. It also offers features like Care Calendar, Well Wishes, and a photo gallery for sharing updates and support—making it easy for volunteers, including those with limited technical skills, to assist. Their website is www.lotsahelpinghands.com.

- **Facebook**
  Facebook is another way to keep your world apprised of what's going on. To keep your cancer-related posts from going out to your entire Facebook universe, you can create a Facebook group with just the people you want to see your health-related posts.

- **Email List**
  A mailing list is simply a list of email addresses of people with whom you want to share your cancer journey. This

enables you to write as little or as often as you want and then send your message out to everyone on your list with a single click.

By reading this chapter, you've already taken a meaningful step toward creating healthier communication boundaries. It's a delicate balance—wanting to keep loved ones informed while prioritizing your own healing.

Remember, it's OK to shift the focus inward and protect your emotional energy. You have permission to limit your outreach, knowing that your closest supporters will be there when you need them most.

This isn't just about conserving energy for today; it's about building the reserves that will sustain you on the path ahead. Trust yourself to honor your own needs and know that setting these boundaries is a powerful act of self-care. Your healing—both physical and emotional—is your priority.

Chapter 3

Enlist the Help of Loved Ones

"An individual doesn't get cancer, a family does."
—TERRY TEMPEST WILLIAMS, *Refuge*

In those first few weeks, I came to understand that accepting help wasn't a luxury—it was a lifeline. Thrust into a world of unfamiliar terminology and daunting treatment options, I found it nearly impossible to prioritize next steps.

During this chaotic time, family and friends can be one of your greatest resources. But while they may want to help, they often don't know how. Giving them clear roles and direction makes it possible for them to contribute to your healing journey.

How Family and Friends Can Help

While you focus on your healing, here are a few ways your support network can lighten your load:

▶ Conduct Research

When I was first diagnosed, the sheer volume of information I had to navigate felt overwhelming. Thankfully, my family stepped in to help. My sister explored traditional treatments, my brother focused on alternative therapies, and my father—having gone through cancer himself—provided invaluable guidance. This kind of support can make an enormous difference.

While you may want to conduct some of your own research, don't hesitate to ask friends and family to help. If you're comfortable with technology, consider using AI tools to gather information. AI can offer insights across a range of medical fields, but always validate the results with a trusted healthcare professional. If this feels overwhelming, ask a tech-savvy friend or relative to help you.

▶ Accompany You to Doctors' Appointments

Initial medical appointments are an emotionally taxing part of cancer care. That's why it is so important to have someone else in the room with you—to take notes, ask questions, and provide the support you need. Because these meetings are often emotionally charged and a fire hose of information, consider asking your doctor for permission to record the session. That way, once you leave the doctor's office, if you are unclear about anything that was said, you can always listen to your recording and verify.

▶ Escort You to Chemotherapy Sessions

While some chemo is administered orally, it often needs to be given intravenously at a facility. If you fall into the second category, ask a friend or family member to drive you to your appointment or keep you company while you're there. Personally, I didn't mind going alone, though my mother was present for my first chemo and my husband was there for my last.

▶ Organize Meals with Helpful Online Tools

Reduce stress on yourself and your primary caregivers by using free online tools that help family, friends, and neighbors stay organized and ensure you have what you need, when you need it.

- **Meal Train**
  www.mealtrain.com
  A free online tool for coordinating meals, restaurant deliveries, and gift cards for food delivery or local restaurants. Friends and family can also note dietary needs and offer other kinds of help like rides or childcare, all in one place to make supporting a loved one easier and less stressful.

- **Care Calendar**
  www.carecalendar.org
  An easy-to-use site for organizing meals, rides, and other support. Helpful features like email reminders and shared calendars keep everyone on the same page so nothing falls through the cracks.

- **Take Them a Meal**
  www.takethemameal.com
  A scheduling tool that helps friends and family organize home-cooked or restaurant-delivered meals using a simple sign-up calendar that prevents double-booking. Participants can note dietary preferences and ideal delivery times. If someone doesn't have time to cook or deliver in person, meals can also be ordered from the site's partner restaurants.

▶ Deliver Groceries and Meals

- Shop for and deliver groceries.
- Drop off nutritious, ready-to-eat meals.

- Give gift certificates to restaurants that deliver or to meal-delivery services.

▶ Stay in Touch with Thoughtful Cards

While texts and emails are always appreciated, cards reflect that someone took the time to pick it out, handwrite a note, and mail it. It's those extra steps that make receiving a card feel special.

▶ Send Daily Affirmations

Even a simple daily affirmation can offer a moment of calm and hope, reminding your loved one that they're not alone. Small acts of kindness, like these, can make a huge difference. One of the most appreciated gifts that I was able to give my friend Kathy, who lived three thousand miles from me, was a daily affirmation. It didn't take long to send in a text. I had a long list of affirmations on my phone that I could just copy, paste, and send. It only took me a couple of minutes to do, but Kathy always told me how much my affirmations boosted her spirits. As for me, this small gesture enabled me to feel that I could add a ray of hope to my dear friend's day as she battled her brain tumor. For sample affirmations, see Chapter 26: Healing Affirmations.

▶ Keep You Company

- Offer to stay with you if you live alone—and even if you don't.
- Invite you to spend the night occasionally so that you feel like you've "gotten away."

  In between my rounds of chemo, one of my dearest friends invited me to fly from San Francisco to join her and her family at a house they rented in a charming Rhode Island beach town for a week. That week away from what I still call cancer world—feasting, laughing, beaching, and biking—gave my soul the infusion it needed to keep going and to trust that everything was going to be all right.

▶ Plan an Outing

- Picnic
- Afternoon tea
- Museum
- Matinee
- Shopping spree
- Walk in the park

▶ Process Insurance Documents

During my cancer care, I found it nearly impossible to keep up with the constant stream of insurance bills, statements, and correspondence. Just trying to make sense of what we owed—and why—became a constant source of frustration. If you have a friend or family member who can help you stay on top of the paperwork, don't hesitate to ask. For support with the process, see Chapter 15: Organize Medical Bills and Insurance Documents.

▶ Assist with Chores

- Pick up prescriptions
- Clean the house
- Help with laundry
- Do the dishes
- Assist with yardwork
- Run errands
- Put bins out for pickup

▶ Help with Childcare

- Offer to babysit
- Help with homework
- Drive to and from school or activities
- Set up playdates

▶ Assist with Pet Care

- Walk the dog
- Take the dog to the dog park
- Brush or groom the pet
- Take the pet to vet or grooming appointments
- Restock the pet's favorite food

Thoughtful Gift Ideas

When people ask if there is anything you need, here are a few ideas you can share. Unlike the earlier suggestions, which are mostly gifts of time, these gifts require a little money but not a lot of time. If sharing your needs feels uncomfortable, consider taking a photo of these pages to send to those who ask how they can help.

▶ Give Books and Magazines

- A copy of *The Cancer-Fighting Kitchen* cookbook by Rebecca Katz (This was my culinary "Bible" when I was going through treatment.)
- A selection of fiction, memoirs, biographies, nonfiction, mysteries, and the latest bestsellers
- A few magazines that are newsworthy, entertaining, or educational

▶ Provide Practical Help

- A bedside water carafe and glass set
- A pretty water pitcher to promote healthy hydration (If the gift giver lives locally, they might want to include "spa water" fixings of fresh cucumber, lemon, lime, or mint.)
- A journal

- A box of thank-you cards and a roll of stamps
- Payment for a cleaning service
- Food or grocery delivery

▶ Give a Sentimental Gift

- A tiny photo album filled with meaningful photos
- A keepsake box to hold cards, notes, and small mementos

▶ Support Rest and Relaxation

- A gift certificate for a massage or a mani-pedi (manicure and pedicure)
- A gift certificate to a local spa
- A gift certificate for a weekend getaway
- A soft blanket
- A lavender eye pillow
- A sound machine that plays soothing sounds like rainforest, jungle, or ocean surf to promote rest
- A set of aromatherapy oils and a diffuser
- A gift basket filled with bath oils, soaps, bubble bath, body scrub, and body lotion
- A gift basket filled with calming items like herbal teas, honey, a teapot, a tall mug, a candle, and cozy socks

▶ Give Clothing

- A bathrobe
- A sweat suit
- A cozy pair of socks or slippers

▶ Send Fresh Flowers

Nothing perks up a room, or one's spirits, quite like a fresh bouquet of flowers, whether they're from your garden or a local florist. My family even went so far as to have bouquets delivered every month for the first six months after I was diagnosed. This gave me something to look forward to at a time when my future was looking bleak.

▶ Provide Visual Escapes for the Journey

- A list of must-see streaming films and television series
- A subscription to a streaming service

▶ Offer Audio Companions for the Journey

- A pair of wireless earbuds for listening to music, podcasts, or audiobooks while resting at home, sitting in waiting rooms, or getting chemo
- A year's subscription to an online music service like Spotify, Apple Music, or Amazon Music
- A year's subscription to audiobook services such as Audible
- A year's subscription to a meditation, sleep, and relaxation app, such as Calm

---

Friends and family can support you in countless ways during your cancer journey. Whether it's accompanying you to appointments or handling everyday tasks, the more clearly you communicate your needs, the more helpful your support network can be. Don't hesitate to ask. Giving someone a specific role not only eases your burden, it gives them the chance to show up in a way that truly matters.

Accepting help is not a sign of weakness. It's a strategic way to preserve your energy so you can focus on healing. As you embark on your journey, embrace the support around you, rely on your community, and let their collective strength nurture you.

Chapter 4

Learn About Your Diagnosis

"Knowledge is power."
—FRANCIS BACON, *Meditationes Sacrae*

No matter the seriousness of your diagnosis, getting informed early is essential. Accurate information is empowering and will better prepare you for consultations with experts. If you're unable to absorb information about your options, ask others to conduct research and help you process it. If you decide to tackle the research yourself, try to limit it to daytime hours. I made the mistake of doing a lot of my reading before bedtime and found that it interfered with a good night's rest.

Understanding Your Diagnosis

Be cautious when using the internet to research your diagnosis. Many sites have misleading or false information. Choose resources that are free of commercial interests. The most reliable sources are hospitals, universities, and major health organizations.

For help separating good information from misinformation, the National Cancer Institute's website (www.cancer.gov/about-cancer/managing-care/using-trusted-resources) features excellent questions to ask, such as:

- Who is publishing the information, and who paid for or sponsored it? (***Tip:*** Check the About Us or Disclaimers section.)
- Is the original source (e.g., research study or medical journal) identified?
- Who reviewed the information before it was posted? (***Tip:*** Check for credentials such as MD, DO, or PhD.)
- How current is the information, and when was it last reviewed?
- What is the web address? (Generally, you can trust websites that end in ".edu" or ".gov." Sites ending in ".org" and ".com" need to be checked for credibility.)
- If personal information is being asked, how is it being used, and how is your privacy protected?

Trustworthy Cancer Resources

The following institutions are among the most reputable and trustworthy cancer resources in the world. Use them to gather information and develop questions for your first appointments:

- The University of Texas MD Anderson Cancer Center, Houston, TX
  www.mdanderson.org
- Memorial Sloan Kettering Cancer Center, New York, NY
  www.mskcc.org
- Mayo Clinic, Rochester, MN (also in Arizona and Florida)
  www.mayoclinic.org/departments-centers/mayo-clinic-cancer-center

- The Johns Hopkins Hospital, Baltimore, MD
  www.hopkinsmedicine.org/kimmel-cancer-center
- UCLA Jonsson Comprehensive Cancer Center, Los Angeles, CA
  www.uclahealth.org/cancer
- Cleveland Clinic, Cleveland, OH
  https://my.clevelandclinic.org/departments/cancer
- Dana-Farber Cancer Institute, Boston, MA
  www.dana-farber.org

Reliable Bilingual Resources (English and Spanish)

The following websites provide trustworthy health information in English and Spanish to help you make informed decisions about your care and treatment:

- **American Cancer Society**
  www.cancer.org
  The American Cancer Society is a nationwide, community-based, voluntary health organization that offers free programs and services to cancer patients. These include expert information on more than seventy different cancer types, a 24/7/365 live helpline, free lodging near treatment centers, rides to treatment, and more.

- **National Cancer Institute (NCI)**
  www.cancer.gov
  The NCI offers extensive support and resources to help cancer patients understand their diagnosis. It provides comprehensive, authoritative information on a wide range of cancer types, treatment options, and research developments. The NCI also offers information on clinical trials.

- **National Institutes of Health (NIH)**
  www.medlineplus.gov
  MedlinePlus is the NIH's website for newly diagnosed cancer patients and their families and friends. Produced by the National Library of Medicine (NLM), the world's largest medical library, it provides reliable, up-to-date health information about various types of cancer, treatments, and management strategies. Additionally, MedlinePlus connects users with clinical trial information.

- **National Comprehensive Cancer Network (NCCN)**
  www.nccn.org/patientresources/patient-resources
  The NCCN website for patients provides comprehensive, reliable resources specifically designed to help cancer patients and their families make informed decisions about care. The site features easy-to-read guides that explain the same treatment plans healthcare professionals use, but in a format designed for patients. These guides help patients understand their type of cancer, available treatments, and what to expect during care.

Understanding your diagnosis is the first step toward reclaiming control. With the right information and support, you'll be better equipped to ask the right questions, make informed choices, and partner with your medical team to create a treatment plan that aligns with your needs and values. Knowledge truly is power—and with it, you can face the road ahead with clarity and confidence.

Chapter 5

Discover Your Treatment Options

"The art of decision making includes
the art of questioning."
—PEARL ZHU, *Decision Master:
The Art and Science of Decision Making*

At this pivotal point in your cancer journey, building confidence in your treatment plan is essential, as it will shape your interactions and experiences within the medical community. Before making any decisions, take the time to fully understand your options.

I remember how overwhelming it felt when I was first faced with a flood of treatment options, each with its own set of unknowns and potential side effects. The weight of those choices was heavy, and the pressure to make the "right" decision was daunting. If you're feeling the same way, know that you're not alone.

If gathering information feels overwhelming, don't hesitate to ask for support from family or friends. I relied heavily on mine, as I couldn't have navigated all the options alone.

How Cancer Treatment Plans Are Decided

Your treatment plan is rarely based on one doctor's opinion alone. Leading institutions follow evidence-based guidelines and collaborate through interdisciplinary teams to personalize care.

- **National Comprehensive Cancer Network (NCCN) guidelines.** These are broad, comprehensive guidelines that cover a wide range of aspects related to cancer care—from diagnosis and treatment to follow-up care and survivorship. They are regularly updated to incorporate the latest research and clinical best practices.

- **American Society of Clinical Oncology (ASCO) guidelines.** These tend to be more narrowly focused on the clinical aspects of oncology. They provide in-depth recommendations specifically aimed at the practice of medical oncology, such as treatment regimens, management of side effects, and other details directly relevant to practicing oncologists.

- **Consultation among doctors.** Collaboration among specialists is a critical aspect of determining the best treatment for a patient. This often involves discussions within a particular specialty (such as oncology) or between different specialties (like medical oncology, surgical oncology, and radiation oncology).

- **Tumor boards.** In complex cases or when there are multiple viable treatment options, a patient's case may be discussed at a tumor board meeting. This is a multidisciplinary team of various specialists, including medical oncologists, surgical oncologists, radiation oncologists (who oversee radiation treatment), pathologists, radiologists (who interpret scans), nurses, and social workers. The tumor board reviews the patient's information and provides a comprehensive, collective opinion on the best treatment approach.

Together, these frameworks ensure that patient care is thorough, up-to-date, and consensus-driven, aiming to provide the most effective and individualized treatment plan possible.

Factors That Influence Your Treatment Options

- The type of cancer
- The stage of the cancer
- Tests that need to be performed on the tumor to provide more information about it, such as biomarkers or hormone receptors
- Additional tests, such as blood tests, X-rays, other imaging scans, or genetic testing
- Your current state of health
- Any additional medical concerns or diagnoses you might have
- Your personal preferences

Fertility and Cancer Treatment: What You Need to Know

If you're of childbearing age and may want to have children in the future, it's crucial to bring this up with your doctor *before* starting any cancer treatment. Some therapies, including chemotherapy, radiation, and surgery, can affect fertility, sometimes permanently. Unfortunately, these conversations are often overlooked in the rush to begin treatment, but they're time-sensitive and can have lifelong implications.

Ask your doctor for a referral to a fertility specialist right away. Options like egg or sperm preservation, embryo freezing, or ovarian suppression may be available, depending on your diagnosis and treatment plan. Even if you're not sure whether you want children—or aren't ready to decide—having the conversation now keeps the door open for the future.

While You Wait for Test Results: What to Ask Your Doctor

- What type of cancer do I have? If you don't know yet, when will you know?
- What stage is my cancer, and what does this mean? If you don't know yet, when will you know?
- What tests are being done on my tumor that can help provide more information?
- Are there any other tests I need to accurately determine how best to proceed?

The Most Common Cancer Treatment Options

The choice of treatment depends on many factors, and often, several therapies are used in combination.

- **Surgery**
  Cancer surgery is a medical procedure to remove cancerous tumors and surrounding tissue, often used to diagnose, treat, or help prevent the spread of cancer.

- **Chemotherapy**
  Chemotherapy involves the use of drugs that kill rapidly dividing cells. It can be administered orally, intravenously, or in other ways such as injections, topical creams, or direct delivery into a body cavity, depending on the cancer. Chemotherapy can be effective for cancers that have spread.

- **Radiation Therapy**
  This treatment uses high doses of radiation to kill cancer cells and shrink tumors by damaging their DNA. It can be delivered externally or internally (brachytherapy).

- **Immunotherapy**
  This is a type of cancer treatment that helps the immune system fight cancer by either boosting the body's natural defenses or using synthetic immune system proteins that help the body recognize and attack cancer cells.

- **Targeted Therapy**
  This treatment precisely identifies and attacks cancer cells, usually while doing minimal damage to normal cells. It uses drugs and other substances that target specific genes or proteins involved in cancer growth.

- **Hormone Therapy**
  Hormone therapy involves blocking or removing hormones that fuel the growth of certain cancers, including breast and prostate cancer. This can be done through medications or surgery.

- **Stem Cell (Bone Marrow) Transplant**
  This involves replacing damaged or diseased bone marrow with healthy stem cells to help the body produce new blood cells and restore the immune system. It is often used after

chemotherapy or radiation for blood-related cancers like leukemia or lymphoma.

- **Precision Medicine**
  This tailors treatment to the individual genetic profiles of patients and their cancer, often using targeted therapies. Precision medicine is a major shift in cancer treatment. It moves away from a one-size-fits-all approach, offering more personalized care that's often more effective and better tolerated by patients. The availability of precision medicine varies widely depending on geographic location, healthcare infrastructure, and the type of cancer. It's more common in developed countries and in settings with advanced healthcare systems.

- **Radiosurgery**
  Radiosurgery is a noninvasive cancer treatment that uses precisely focused, high-dose radiation to target and destroy tumors, often in the brain or spine, without surgical incisions.

- **Cryoablation and Radiofrequency Ablation**
  These are minimally invasive treatments that destroy cancer cells using extreme cold (cryoablation) or heat generated by high-frequency radio waves (radiofrequency ablation).

Where You Can Connect with Others in a Similar Situation

- Check with relatives, friends, neighbors, coworkers, and members of a congregation, club, or other groups you belong to.

- Contact the Cancer Hope Network through their website: www.cancerhopenetwork.org. This organization provides free, confidential support by matching patients with trained volunteers who have had similar cancer experiences. This kind of peer mentorship can offer valuable emotional insight, practical advice, and a sense of connection through shared experiences.
- Research local cancer support groups.
- Explore online cancer communities, discussion boards, and forums.
- Get connected with someone who has the same type of cancer as you through a cancer association.
- Ask your hospital or cancer center if they can match you with a group or volunteer.

Questions You Should Ask Your Mentor or Group

- What do you know now that you wish you had known earlier?
- What websites, social media, or online groups have you found most valuable?
- What other forms of support have you found to be helpful?
- What side effects did you experience, and how did you manage them?
- Do you know anyone else who has navigated this kind of cancer?

Though this journey is challenging, taking the time to understand your options—however overwhelming that may feel—empowers you to approach each decision with greater confidence. With the support of loved ones and a growing understanding of your choices, you'll be better prepared to make decisions that truly align with your personal needs and values.

Each thoughtful choice brings you closer to a path that's truly your own.

PART TWO

SET YOURSELF UP FOR SUCCESS

Chapter 6

Be Your Own Advocate

"It is not in the stars to hold our destiny, but in ourselves."
—WILLIAM SHAKESPEARE, *Julius Caesar*

A cancer diagnosis can feel like a surreal slap in the face, no matter who you are. While you may feel you've lost control over how your life is going to unfold, adopting a take-charge approach will play a critical role in your health and healing. Advocating for yourself doesn't mean being difficult—it means respecting your needs and ensuring your voice is part of every decision. If you're not up to being your own advocate, then find someone who can be. Either way, ensure you get the best possible care by trusting your judgment and sharing your questions and concerns.

Trust Your Gut

Diagnosed with an aggressive cancer at a relatively young age—and with no family history of breast cancer—I couldn't help but wonder why I had gotten this dreaded disease. Shortly after my diagnosis, I was put in touch with the sister of one of my husband's colleagues. It turned out that she had found herself in a similar situation just a year earlier. She advised me that if I had any Ashkenazi Jewish ancestors—which I did—I should get genetically tested for the BRCA gene before deciding how to proceed.

BRCA stands for "BReast CAncer" gene—mutations in BRCA1 or BRCA2 significantly increase the risk of breast and ovarian cancers.

After completing a detailed questionnaire at UCSF's Genetic Testing Center, my counselor strongly discouraged me from getting tested. Based on my answers, she thought that there was little to no chance I carried the gene.

My gut told me otherwise. So I got the test. When I returned to UCSF weeks later to get the results, I was greeted by my genetic counselor, who asked if I was sure I wanted to know. At that moment, I knew I had tested positive for the gene and that there was a fifty-fifty chance I had passed it on to my son.

A positive test result means that you have a mutation in one of the breast cancer genes, BRCA1 or BRCA2, and therefore a much higher risk of developing breast or ovarian cancer compared to someone without the mutation. However, a positive result doesn't mean you're certain to develop cancer.

Considering the weight of a positive test result, I requested that a second test be sent to a different lab to verify the findings. Once the second test also came back positive, I knew what I had to do. Unfortunately, my breasts, ovaries, and fallopian tubes all had to go.

In the end, these precautionary measures may very well have saved my life.

Don't Be Intimidated by Your Doctor

The person overseeing your cancer care should be someone whose opinion you trust and whose demeanor puts you at ease. Your meetings may be brief, but you should always feel seen and heard by your doctor. Remember, the best doctors are still human, and mistakes happen—which is just one of the reasons your voice matters. If your doctor isn't listening, explaining clearly, or showing the compassion you need, don't hesitate to speak up.

If Your Oncologist Doesn't Instill Confidence, Find Another

About a week before I was to have my mastectomy, I serendipitously ran into my radiologist. To ensure that I would be well protected during my surgery, she asked if I had upped my intake of my antiestrogen medication. At the time, I was on toremifene, which I had chosen over tamoxifen because my research showed it generally caused fewer side effects. Tamoxifen, while effective, can increase the risk of blood clots, stroke, and endometrial cancer.[1]

My radiologist explained that I should have increased my toremifene dose for the ten days leading up to surgery—something my oncologist had failed to mention. She emphasized this wasn't just a minor slipup. It was a serious oversight. That ten-day lead time was critical for the medication to reach therapeutic levels, suppress hormone-sensitive cancer cells, and potentially lower the risk of recurrence during and after surgery. Fortunately, I still had almost a week to ramp up the medication, but once I fully grasped the gravity of the situation, my confidence in my oncologist's judgment was deeply shaken.

It was clear I needed a new oncologist, so I asked the women in my support group to share who had earned their confidence. Only a few hands went up—and every single one pointed to the same doctor. After learning more about Dr. Newman, I couldn't wait to meet him. When I did, I was reassured that I was under the best of care. Not only was he incredibly competent, but he also had a great bedside manner, never letting me leave his office without answering all my questions. He was definitely the gold standard.

Stand Your Ground

The day before my bilateral mastectomy, I met with my surgeon in San Francisco to go over last-minute details. At the eleventh hour, she tried to talk me out of the deep inferior epigastric perforator (DIEP) flap reconstructive surgery, a procedure I had already committed to both emotionally and intellectually.

At the time, the DIEP flap was an advanced and relatively uncommon technique that preserved the abdominal muscle. It used only fat, skin, and blood vessels from the lower belly, which were microsurgically reattached to the chest. By contrast, the more widely used transverse rectus abdominis myocutaneous (TRAM) flap involved cutting through the abdominal wall muscle, often leading to a longer recovery and more complications. But the greatest risk for me wasn't medical at all. A TRAM flap might have taken from me the ability to lift and hold my toddler—a bond I needed as much as he did.

My surgeon shared three concerns: She preferred the more familiar TRAM flap, favored same-day reconstruction, and worried I'd have to wait nearly seven months for the DIEP procedure. This would have left me with deflated breasts for more than half a year—a reality I didn't easily embrace either. But deep down, I knew it was the right decision for me.

As soon as I left her office, I called my reconstructive surgeon in New Orleans and insisted he speak with her immediately—a conversation that should have happened long before. The next day, when I arrived for surgery, it was delayed by several hours. I later discovered that barely an hour before the procedure, my reconstructive surgeon had faxed detailed drawings to my surgeon, illustrating how she should cut my breasts to optimize the reconstruction. So, while I sat anxiously in pre-op, my surgeon was studying those diagrams with her team. I can't help but wonder what would have happened had I not made that call.

Placing that call was an intuitive decision—one I knew could change everything. Trusting my voice made the difference between a good outcome and a disaster. In that moment, I almost felt like the person behind the curtain, pulling the levers to ensure everything went according to plan. It felt strangely powerful to know I was making sure all the pieces fell into place. That sense of control—knowing I was orchestrating my own care—gave me confidence when I needed it most.

Considerations for Surgery at a Teaching Hospital

Another aspect of self-advocacy is knowing what to expect if your care takes place in a teaching hospital.

Cancer care at a teaching hospital has several major benefits, including access to the latest medical advancements and innovative treatment options. That said, it's important to understand what a teaching hospital is to make sure it aligns with your expectations.

In teaching hospitals, medical residents and fellows often perform surgeries as part of their hands-on training. While you benefit from a collaborative team of medical professionals, as a patient, you have the right to request that the attending surgeon you personally selected perform your surgery. If your medical circumstances are particularly complex, communicating this preference in advance can help set clear expectations.

At the same time, it's worth recognizing that teaching hospitals play an essential role in educating the next generation of surgeons. The involvement of residents and fellows, under the supervision of experienced physicians, is a critical component of their training. While patients often benefit from their participation—through added oversight and access to the latest knowledge—it's important to remember that you have the right to be clear about your expectations.

Get to Know Your Support Team

If you want to get the attention you need and deserve, it is important that you establish a good rapport with all the members of your cancer care team. Since many of them will be spending more time with you than your doctor, they are in a better position to help you day in and day out.

Take a moment to understand the specific roles of each team member, whether it's the nurse navigator, social worker, nutritionist, or oncology nurse. Knowing the right person to contact for specific concerns, such as medication side effects or dietary issues, will help make your care more effective.

To enlist your team members' support, always be kind and take the time to ask each member the best way to reach them, whether it's by voicemail, email, or your patient portal. Keep their information close at hand. Ask about how quickly you can expect to hear back. This will help you manage your expectations and reduce stress.

Building personal connections is also key. Get to know your team members by name and take note of their individual personalities. This small gesture can help create a more collaborative and invested relationship.

Whenever possible, keep a log of important conversations and messages with your care team. Having a record of instructions or advice can help you stay organized and avoid misunderstandings. If keeping track is overwhelming, consider asking a friend or loved one to help, or use a dedicated notebook or app to capture key details.

Be proactive, but patient. While it's important to advocate for yourself, it's also essential to approach your team with patience and understanding. Remember, they are managing many patients at once.

Lastly, remember to express gratitude when your team goes the extra mile. Even the simplest "thank you" can strengthen your bond with those supporting you.

Advocating for yourself is an act of self-respect. No matter how overwhelming the process may seem, remember that you are not powerless.

Being your own advocate doesn't mean being adversarial; it means honoring yourself—asking questions, challenging opinions, and trusting your instincts, even in the face of resistance. Valuing your own voice and standing firm in your decisions matters, because no one understands your needs better than you. In the end, advocating for yourself isn't just a strategy—it's an expression of your inner strength and one of the most powerful steps you can take on the road to healing.

Chapter 7

Request the Expertise of Patient Navigators

"No man is wise enough by himself."
—PLAUTUS, *Trinummus*

Patient navigators are trained professionals who help ease your healthcare journey by guiding you to the medical and supportive services you need. Their presence in cancer care facilities reflects a patient-centered approach, increasingly recognized as crucial for improving clinical outcomes and patient satisfaction.[1]

Cancer centers that offer patient navigator services generally find that these programs contribute to patient outcomes in several key areas:

- Increased screening and diagnostic follow-up
- Enhanced treatment adherence
- Reduced delays in care
- Improved patient satisfaction

- Better health outcomes
- Reduction in healthcare disparities

During my cancer treatment in 2002, I lacked the support of a patient navigator. Fortunately, patient navigators are now becoming increasingly accessible at large hospitals and comprehensive cancer centers across the country. Today, patients are discovering the emotional, financial, and logistical advantages of collaborating with a patient navigator through every phase of their cancer journey.

Patient navigators can be healthcare professionals—usually nurses or social workers—or nonclinical members of the community. For example, nurse navigators may assist patients with symptom management, while other navigators help ensure continuity of care by assisting with logistics. These navigators are there to guide you in many ways throughout treatment, offering support that includes:

- **Care coordination.** Care coordinators help manage the logistics of cancer treatment: scheduling appointments, arranging referrals, and ensuring you connect with the right specialists. They also translate complex medical language into understandable terms so you can make informed decisions.

- **Emotional and social support.** Navigators offer emotional support and can connect you with counseling services, support groups, translators, and transportation to medical appointments. They also provide coaching to enhance patient-doctor communication and offer social service support if your treatment impacts housing or food security.

- **Financial and insurance assistance.** Resource coordinators help you understand your insurance benefits and out-of-pocket costs and can guide you through the complexities of insurance claims. They can also connect you with financial aid resources and programs that help cover treatment and medication costs.

- **Educational resources.** Support specialists offer trusted information about your diagnosis, treatment options, and potential side effects. This helps you make informed decisions about your care.

- **Advocacy.** Healthcare liaisons advocate for you with healthcare providers, ensuring your concerns are addressed and your preferences respected. They also help facilitate communication among members of your healthcare team.

- **Follow-up and continuity of care.** Cancer care coordinators help manage follow-up appointments and transitions between different stages of treatment, making sure no part of your care gets lost in the shuffle.

- **Holistic and integrative resources.** Patient navigators can also introduce you to holistic and integrative health approaches that complement your medical treatments. These may include nutrition, exercise, and mind-body therapies, which can enhance your overall well-being during treatment.

In an ideal world, patient navigators are involved in your care as early as the screening process. Sometimes, multiple navigators may assist a patient at different stages of their journey. For example, one navigator might help you take the next steps after an abnormal screening test, while another might guide you after receiving your diagnosis.

Historically, patient navigation services have been inconsistent because they have primarily relied on funding from foundations, donations, and medical institutions. However, at the time of this writing, recent changes—such as the Biden Cancer Moonshot program—have enabled the Centers for Medicare & Medicaid Services (CMS) to implement new rules for 2024 that reimburse patient navigation services. This makes it easier for cancer centers and local clinics to offer these services to everyone, especially for those who might otherwise face barriers to timely, effective care.

Private health insurers are also beginning to cover patient navigation services in response to President Joe Biden's initiative. This trend is driven by studies showing that these services help manage chronic diseases, improve treatment adherence and outcomes, and reduce hospital readmissions, ultimately lowering costs for insurers.

For optimal care, I recommend beginning your journey by finding a patient navigator. You can learn about these services through the following resources:

- Your oncologist
- Your primary care doctor
- The patient services department at your cancer center
- Your health insurance provider
- Support groups

Nonprofit organizations can also provide valuable support and resources to help you navigate your treatment and care. Notable nonprofits include American Cancer Society, Cancer Support Community, Susan G. Komen, Blood Cancer United (formerly The Leukemia & Lymphoma Society, or LLS), Patient Advocate Foundation, and Livestrong Foundation. For specific details on how to access these services, it's best to visit their websites or contact them directly.

You don't have to do this alone.

Ultimately, a patient navigator can be a critical ally on your cancer journey, offering not just logistical support but also emotional guidance, advocacy, and a sense of partnership when you need it most. Whether you're newly diagnosed or entering a new phase of treatment, ask your care team about connecting with a navigator. Their support can simplify decisions and ensure you get the care you deserve.

Chapter 8

Assemble the Best Possible Medical Team

"Alone we can do so little; together we can do so much."
—HELEN KELLER, attributed to her
vaudeville performances, c. 1920s

Building the right medical team is one of the most crucial steps you'll take after a cancer diagnosis. The quality of your care often hinges on the expertise, communication, and collaboration of the specialists guiding your treatment. Over the course of my treatment, I assembled and collaborated with a team of a dozen medical professionals and six integrative care specialists.

I had a solid track record for choosing excellent doctors, but not all of them made it to the finish line with me. To pass my litmus test, my doctors needed a strong reputation, clinical expertise, an affiliation with a well-respected medical center, empathy, respect for my point of view, and ideally an appreciation for complementary healing modalities.

Managing chemo, radiation, and five surgeries over several years wasn't easy, but I was always surrounded by the care and expertise of my handpicked team. That made all the difference in the world.

When assembling your team, it's important to remember that finding the right professionals isn't just about medical credentials—it's about identifying the doctors, treatment centers, and support systems that align with your needs and values. Sometimes, cancer patients choose where they want to be treated before they choose who they want to be treated by. It's important to think about how the environment, resources, and philosophy of a treatment center can contribute to your well-being.

How to Choose the Right Cancer Treatment Center

If possible, consider choosing an oncologist at a teaching hospital, meaning one that is affiliated with a medical school. Here you will find:

- Improved quality of care
- Specialists in your type of cancer
- Access to new cures and treatment therapies
- Opportunities to explore clinical trials
- State-of-the-art technologies
- Shorter hospital stays for major illnesses
- Superior outcomes and survival rates
- Specialized surgeries and experimental medical procedures

To find cancer facilities that deliver cutting-edge treatments, visit the National Cancer Institute-Designated Cancer Centers' website: www.cancer.gov/research/infrastructure/cancer-centers/find.

How to Find an Oncologist

After receiving a cancer diagnosis, finding the right oncologist is one of the most important decisions you'll make. Oncologists are medical doctors who specialize in diagnosing, treating, and managing cancer. There are several types of oncologists, each focusing on different aspects of cancer treatment: medical oncologists, surgical oncologists, radiation oncologists, pediatric oncologists, and hematologist oncologists, who specialize in blood cancers such as leukemia and lymphoma. All these specialists work together to provide comprehensive care to patients.

Start by looking for an oncologist with extensive experience treating your specific type of cancer. Don't be shy about asking how many patients with your cancer type they treat each year. You are entitled to this information so you can make the best possible choice for your care.

If you are feeling overwhelmed right now, I completely understand. This process can feel daunting. But each step you take brings you closer to the care team you deserve.

STEP 1: Cast a Wide Net

- Ask your primary care physician, "If I were your sister (or brother), who would you recommend that I see at (your preferred institution)?"
- Enlist your community to help you identify and secure appointments with the best Western physicians. Consider also seeking advice from integrative doctors, whose holistic and complementary approach focuses on your physical, emotional, mental, social, and spiritual well-being. My work with Dr. Keith Block, a Chicago-based pioneer and leader in integrative cancer care, enhanced my care and was key to my healing success.

- Seek personal connections to renowned medical facilities or oncologists that specialize in your type of cancer, even beyond your inner circle. Spread the word far and wide via email, text, and social media, if appropriate. Give your contacts permission to forward your message to others who might be able to help.
- Talk to people in your area who are currently undergoing cancer treatment or who may know someone who is. They are likely to be good sources of information about trusted doctors and facilities in your medical community.
- Online cancer communities are another great resource for identifying which centers are most active in treating and researching your specific cancer type.
- If you don't have a personal referral to a busy doctor, call their office and ask for the new patient coordinator. These staff members are often nurses whose job is to provide an expedited path to appointments.
- Advocate fiercely for the quality care you deserve. If you are unable to find a local expert, search elsewhere. You can often visit an oncologist in a different city or state and still receive treatment locally. If traveling is cost-prohibitive, refer to the Financial Resources section in the back of this book. You'd be surprised how many free or low-cost options are available to cancer patients.

STEP 2: Get a Referral

Once you find a doctor who meets your criteria, call the office to find out if they accept your insurance. If they do, call your primary doctor's office and ask them to make a referral. This "referral rule" is all about insurance coverage. That's why most doctors won't schedule an appointment or speak with you until they have received a referral from your primary care physician.

STEP 3: Send Medical Records *Before* Making Your Appointment

Once the referral has been sent, make sure your primary care physician's office sends your medical records. In almost all cases, doctors won't let you make an appointment until they've already received your records and read through your file.

Questions to Help You Evaluate Doctors

Bring the same list of questions to all your doctor appointments so that you can easily compare. At the top of each sheet, include:

- The doctor's name
- Who referred you
- Any relevant notes about the doctor's reputation

After each appointment, jot down your answers to the following:

- Is this someone whose judgment you can trust?
- Did you feel seen and heard during your appointment?
- What did you like most about this doctor?
- What did you like least about this doctor?
- Is this the person you want to lead your cancer care team?

When choosing a doctor, try not to focus solely on bedside manner. While it's preferable to feel camaraderie, the most important factor is whether you trust their judgment and feel confident in their care.

Don't Overlook the Third Option

While traveling on the Marin Airporter several years ago, I overheard two women trying to solve a problem that seemed to elude them both.

Then one of the women blurted out, "Well, there's always the third option."

Her friend looked confused. "What third option?"

She could hardly wait to reveal her secret: "It's the one you don't know about yet!"

The same goes for cancer care. If you're feeling conflicted about which doctor to choose, which protocol to follow, or whether to commit to a nearby medical facility or a renowned teaching hospital that requires a lengthy commute, remember that there's likely a third option. My third option was ultimately to take the advice of the top breast cancer oncologist at UCSF (a two-hour round-trip commute) and have her protocol implemented at a cancer facility close to home.

Chapter 9

Make the Most of Medical Appointments

"In the fields of observation,
chance favors only the prepared mind."
—LOUIS PASTEUR, inaugural lecture at
the University of Lille, December 7, 1854

Your first medical appointments can feel overwhelming, but they also offer an important opportunity: to take charge of your care. A little preparation goes a long way in making these visits more productive and less intimidating.

After my diagnosis, I took this advice seriously. My family used to joke that I needed a small wagon to haul around my giant three-ring binder. As time went on, it became a portable archive of my entire medical history, packed with everything from pathology reports and imaging results to detailed Q&As for every doctor's appointment. I wasn't leaving anything to chance!

Making the Most of Your Appointment Time

When scheduling, ask how much time has been allocated for your visit. This will help you set realistic expectations and organize your questions. To make the most of your time, let your doctor know early on what you hope to cover. For example, you might begin by saying, "We have a few important questions we'd like to cover. When would be the best time to go through them?" Setting the stage like this helps ensure that your concerns are addressed and that your time together is as productive as possible.

What to Bring to Your Initial Appointments

▶ Completed Forms

Your cancer care facility will likely provide a variety of forms that need to be completed before you arrive at your first appointment. Find out if they need to be submitted ahead of time or if you should turn them in at your appointment.

▶ Medical Profile

If you didn't receive forms to complete before your appointment, prepare a one- to two-page document summarizing all relevant information about your medical history to bring with you for your healthcare providers. To make updating and duplicating easy, enter all this data into a computer. If you are unable to do this yourself, ask someone to help. While it may require some effort upfront, it will save you a significant amount of time in the long run by preventing the need to repeatedly remember the same details. At the top of your medical profile, include your name, address, phone number, email, birth date, and blood type, then enter the following:

- Health insurance information
- Healthcare team contact information
- Personal health history, including current conditions, diseases, medical events, surgeries, and hospitalizations, as well as the year and medical center for each
- Results of any genetic testing for cancer (such as BRCA1, BRCA2, or other hereditary cancer panels)
- Family health history, including family history of cancer (types of cancer, age at diagnosis, or multiple cancers in one person); genetic disorders linked to cancer; ethnicity and ancestry; reproductive health issues, such as endometriosis or early menopause; and autoimmune disorders (This is important for assessing potential genetic risks and tailoring screening and treatment strategies.)
- List of current medications, dosage, frequency, prescription start date, reason prescribed, and prescribing doctor
- List of any supplements and herbs, along with dosages
- List of drug allergies and your body's reaction to each
- Emergency contact name, phone number, and relationship

▶ A Friend or Family Member

Newly diagnosed cancer patients can all benefit from bringing a loved one to their initial doctors' appointments. When emotions run high, it's harder to absorb complex medical information. That's why it is important to be accompanied by someone who can not only offer moral support but also take notes for you and ask questions you may not think to ask.

▶ Sample Questions to Ask Your Medical Oncologist

- How serious is my diagnosis?
- What stage is my cancer and what does that mean?
- What treatment options do you recommend and why?

- What is the goal of my treatment (e.g., remission, prolonging life, symptom management)?
- What are the most serious side effects that I can expect from each treatment option?
- How soon should I start treatment?
- How many cases like mine have you treated?
- What happens if my cancer doesn't respond to the current treatment?
- Is there a clinical trial happening that I would qualify to participate in?
- How will this treatment impact my quality of life?
- What lifestyle or dietary changes should I consider during treatment?

▶ Sample Questions to Ask Your Surgical Oncologist

- What is the goal of the surgery in my case?
- What type of surgery will I need, and why is it the best option for me?
- How critical is the timing of this procedure?
- What are the risks and potential complications of this surgery?
- Are there any immediate or long-term side effects I should be aware of?
- What will my recovery process look like, and how long will it take?
- What can I expect regarding pain management after the surgery?
- How will this surgery impact my daily life and activities?
- What are the chances of cancer recurrence after this surgery?
- What follow-up care will be necessary after the surgery?

▶ Sample Questions to Ask Your Radiation Oncologist

- What is the goal of radiation therapy in my case?
- What type of radiation therapy will I receive and why?

- How long will my treatment last and how many sessions will I need?
- How will we monitor the effectiveness of the treatment?
- What lifestyle or dietary changes should I consider during treatment?
- How can I manage or mitigate side effects during and after treatment?
- Will radiation therapy affect my other medications or treatments?
- Will I need to take time off work, and for how long?
- What support services are available to help me during treatment?

Sample Questions to Ask Your Pediatric Oncologist

- How many children with this type of cancer have you treated?
- Are you specialized in treating specific types of pediatric cancers?
- What are the most effective treatment options available for my child's specific condition?
- How will the treatment affect my child's growth and development?
- What are the potential short- and long-term side effects of the proposed treatments?
- How can we manage or mitigate these side effects?
- Are there support groups or resources for children and families going through similar treatments?
- How do you involve parents in the decision-making process?
- How often will my child need to come in for checkups or scans?

Sample Questions to Ask Your Hematologist Oncologist

- How frequently do you treat patients with my specific type of hematologic condition or cancer?

- What is your experience with the latest treatment advancements for my condition?
- Can you explain my diagnosis in detail and outline the available treatment options?
- What are the potential benefits and risks of each treatment option?
- How will you monitor the effectiveness of the treatment over time?
- What signs should I look for that might indicate a need to adjust my treatment plan?
- What are the possible side effects of the treatment and how can they be managed?
- Are there any lifestyle or dietary changes I should consider to help manage my condition?
- How will you coordinate care with other specialists, such as cardiologists or endocrinologists, if necessary?
- Will you work with my primary care physician to ensure comprehensive care?

▶ A Phone to Record Your Appointment (with Your Doctor's Permission)

Recording conversations at doctors' appointments will help you keep track of medical information that may be presented to you faster than you can process in real time. If your doctor is unwilling to let you record the appointment, consider it a red flag. Clear communication and transparency are essential to your care. When you get home, if you have time, I highly recommend that you transcribe the recording (or at least the key content). I always found that I could wrap my head around the information better when I could see it. If you don't have time to do this, you can still benefit from listening to the recording and jotting down any questions that arise.

What to Bring to Follow-Up Appointments

▶ A List of Questions

- Make your questions specific and brief.
- Number your questions by order of importance, as your time with the doctor will be limited.
- Request to see any relevant visual records, such as:
    - X-rays
    - CT scans (computed tomography)
    - MRIs (magnetic resonance imaging)
    - PET scans (positron emission tomography)
    - Ultrasound images
    - Mammograms
    - Pathology slides
    - Bone scans
    - Surgical diagrams
    - Radiation treatment plans
    - Genetic test results

Seeing these can make complex information easier to understand. If they aren't available during your appointment, ask if they can be provided later. For example, "If some of these images aren't available now, could they be sent to me or shown at my next appointment?"

▶ Side Effects Journal

If you are experiencing discomfort from your illness, treatment, or medications, it's crucial for your medical team to have specific details about your symptoms. Keeping a journal can help. Bring this journal to your appointments so you don't have to rely on memory. If you use an app for journaling, consider printing your entries since the last visit and emailing them to your doctor or sending them through your facility's portal before your next appointment.

Consider including the following in your journal:

- List of side effects
- Date and time of each side effect
- Potential cause of each side effect
- Duration of each side effect
- Intensity of each side effect on a scale of 0 to 10, with 10 being the worst
- Impact of each side effect on daily activities, such as eating, sleeping, working, walking, exercising, and sexual intimacy

---

You now have the tools and strategies to make the most of your medical appointments and build a strong relationship with your care team. Each meeting is an opportunity to get the answers you need, clarify your treatment options, and ensure that your voice is heard. Remember, being prepared and proactive is more than just a strategy; it's a way to regain a sense of control and actively participate in your healing journey.

Chapter 10

Seek Second Opinions

> "It is the mark of an educated mind to be able to entertain a thought without accepting it."
> —ARISTOTLE, *Metaphysics*

Seeking multiple perspectives on your diagnosis isn't just wise—it could be lifesaving. Each doctor brings their own expertise and approach, and a second opinion can uncover treatment options you hadn't considered—or affirm that you're on the right path.

When I was first diagnosed, I consulted with three different oncologists: one from Stanford, another from UCSF, and a third at a local cancer center. Each opinion added a layer of understanding and provided me with the confidence to make informed decisions about my treatment plan. When looking for a specialist, seek someone who has extensive experience in your specific type of cancer. This could be a medical oncologist, surgical oncologist, or radiation oncologist, depending on your needs.

If you're near a large city, opt for hospitals with medical specialists and surgeons who are likely to have more advanced training than those at smaller local hospitals. If you live in a more remote area, consider telemedicine. Many top cancer centers offer video and phone consultations, enabling you to access world experts from the comfort of your home.

Check Your Insurance Coverage Before Scheduling Second-Opinion Appointments

To protect yourself financially, review your insurance policy or contact your provider to understand your coverage for second opinions.

- **Standard coverage.** Most insurance plans cover one second opinion, especially for significant diagnoses such as cancer. This coverage is often included to ensure that patients receive the most accurate diagnosis and appropriate treatment plan.

- **Additional opinions.** Coverage for more than one second opinion can vary. Some plans might cover additional opinions if the first and second opinions differ significantly or if the patient requests further clarification.

- **Network providers.** Insurance companies may require that the second opinion come from a provider within their network. Going out-of-network could lead to higher out-of-pocket costs for the patient.

- **Pre-authorization.** Some insurance plans require pre-authorization before they will cover the cost of a second opinion. Check with your insurance company to understand the requirements and ensure that a second opinion will be covered.

- **Specific conditions.** For certain conditions, such as cancer, insurance plans may have more flexible policies and might cover multiple second opinions due to the complexity and seriousness of the disease.

Questions to Ask at Your Appointment

When seeking a second opinion, you should ask a variety of questions to gain a comprehensive understanding of your diagnosis and treatment options. Here are some key questions to consider:

▶ Diagnosis and Pathology

- Can you review my pathology report and explain it to me?
- Can your pathology team examine and evaluate my biopsy to verify the diagnosis?
  (Often, you will have to sign a release for one medical center to send the biopsy specimen to another.)
- Is the type and stage of my cancer accurately identified?
- Are there any additional tests or biopsies you recommend?

▶ Treatment Options

- What are all the treatment options available for my type and stage of cancer?
- What treatment do you recommend, and why?
- Are there alternative treatments that I should consider?
- What are the goals of the recommended treatment (curative, palliative, etc.)?

▶ Risks and Benefits

- What are the potential benefits and risks of each treatment option?

- What are the possible side effects, and how can they be managed?
- How might the treatments impact my daily life and activities?

▶ Expertise and Experience

- How many patients with my type of cancer have you treated?
- What is your experience with the recommended treatments?

▶ Clinical Trials

- Are there any clinical trials available for my type of cancer?
- Would I be a candidate for any of these trials?

▶ Prognosis and Outcomes

- What is the expected prognosis with the recommended treatment?
- How do the different treatment options affect my prognosis?

▶ Logistics and Practicalities

- How often and for how long will I need to undergo treatment?
- Where will the treatments take place?

▶ Support and Resources

- What support services are available for me and my family?
- Can you refer me to other specialists or resources for additional support?

▶ Follow-Up Care

- What is the follow-up plan after treatment?
- How will my response to treatment be monitored?

▶ Next Steps

- How do your recommendations compare to those of my initial doctor?
- Would you be willing to coordinate with my current care team?

By asking these questions, you can gather detailed information that will help you make informed decisions about your treatment options and overall care plan.

How Patient Records Are Managed and Shared

Many cancer specialists require a review of all medical records before agreeing to a consultation. Fortunately, it has never been easier to share your medical records. Modern medical centers use Electronic Health Record (EHR) systems to securely share patient information, such as medical history, test results, imaging, and treatment plans, so everyone involved in your care stays connected and informed. Practices can vary, so check with your healthcare providers to understand how your records are managed and shared.

In addition to provider-to-provider portals, many medical centers offer patient portals. These allow you to access your own medical records, view test results, communicate with your healthcare team, and, in some cases, authorize the sharing of your records with other providers.

For your own peace of mind, maintain copies of all medical records, including test results, pathology reports, imaging studies, and treatment plans. Keep these records easily accessible and bring them to second-opinion appointments. This ensures your information is readily available when needed.

Choosing the right treatment path can feel overwhelming, but each second opinion is a step toward making the most informed decisions for your health. Seeking multiple perspectives isn't just about confirming a diagnosis, it's about empowering yourself with knowledge, building confidence in your choices, and finding the approach that's right for you. Trust that every step you take, whether it confirms your current direction or opens new possibilities, is part of honoring yourself and prioritizing your well-being.

Chapter 11

Find Out If a Clinical Trial Is Right for You

"There is no medicine like hope, no incentive so great, and no tonic so powerful as expectation of something tomorrow."
—ORISON SWETT MARDEN, *Pushing to the Front*

A clinical trial is a research study conducted with human participants to evaluate the safety, effectiveness, and potential side effects of new medical interventions, such as drugs, devices, treatments, or diagnostic procedures. Such trials are essential for both developing and validating new treatments and ensuring their safety for broader use. They are meticulously designed and regulated to uphold ethical standards and protect participant safety.

Before considering a clinical trial, it's important to first discuss your options with your healthcare provider. They can help determine whether a clinical trial is appropriate for your specific condition, guide you through the potential risks and benefits, and ensure that your decision aligns with your overall treatment plan. This collaborative approach empowers you to make informed choices and feel more confident about the path you choose.

Personally, when I was facing stage 3 cancer, I chose not to participate in a clinical trial because I wasn't comfortable with the risks. For me, the unknowns—like unexpected side effects or the chance of receiving a placebo—felt too significant, outweighing any potential benefits the trial might have offered. While clinical trials are essential for advancing treatments, it's important for each person to weigh the pros and cons based on their own circumstances and comfort level.

Phases of Clinical Trials

Every new cancer treatment must go through a careful process of testing. Clinical trials are carried out in four phases, each designed to answer different questions about safety and effectiveness:

- **PHASE I.** Tests a treatment in a small group of participants to find the safest dose and identify potential side effects. In cancer trials, these participants are often patients who have already undergone standard treatments and may have advanced or treatment-resistant disease.

- **PHASE II.** Studies a larger group to evaluate how well the treatment works while continuing to monitor safety.

- **PHASE III.** Expands to an even larger group to confirm effectiveness, track side effects, and compare the new treatment with standard options.

- **PHASE IV.** Follows a treatment after approval to gather more information on its safety and effectiveness in broader populations and tracks long-term side effects.

As participants move through these phases, they may continue in the trial or exit, depending on the results. If a treatment causes serious side effects or proves ineffective, the trial may be paused or stopped. Conversely, if the treatment shows promise, participants might transition from one phase to the next, sometimes alongside newly enrolled participants.

The outcomes of clinical trials are essential in developing new medical treatments and expanding medical knowledge. Still, success in a clinical trial doesn't always lead to immediate regulatory approval or widespread availability. Even after positive results, it can take years for a treatment to gain full approval and become accessible to patients.

Considerations When Enrolling in a Clinical Trial

For some cancer patients, enrolling in a clinical trial may be a valuable option, offering early access to promising new therapies. However, each clinical trial has its own benefits and risks.

▶ Potential Benefits

- **Access to new treatments.** Participants may receive cutting-edge treatments before they become widely available.

- **Close monitoring.** Regular and careful attention by qualified professionals can lead to better overall care during the trial.

- **Cost coverage.** Some trials may cover the cost of treatment, travel, and other related expenses.

- **Contribution to research.** Participation helps advance medical research, potentially benefiting future patients. The breast cancer treatments we have today, including Herceptin, tamoxifen, aromatase inhibitors, and taxanes, are available thanks to the many women who participated in clinical trials to test them.

- **Active role in care.** Many participants feel empowered by taking an active role in their treatment, which can lead to a more positive outlook and better quality of life.

▶ Potential Risks

- **Randomization.** In randomized trials, participants are assigned to treatment groups by chance and may receive a placebo, which is an inactive substance or treatment that has no therapeutic effect. The placebo is used to help researchers determine if the new treatment is truly effective compared to no treatment at all. However, this also means that participants might not receive the active medication or treatment, which could impact their outcomes.

- **Ineffectiveness.** The new treatment may not work for everyone and could be less effective than existing options.

- **Side effects.** Experimental treatments may have unknown or severe side effects.

- **Insurance issues.** Not all trial-related costs may be covered by insurance.

- **Increased testing.** Clinical trials often require frequent visits and tests, leading to more time spent in medical facilities.

Finding and Participating in a Clinical Trial[1]

Here are the steps you should follow when trying to find and participate in a clinical trial:

STEP 1: Consult with Your Doctor

- **Discuss options.** Talk to your primary care doctor or specialist about clinical trials relevant to your condition.

- **Get recommendations.** Ask for their opinion on whether participating in a clinical trial is a good option for you and if they know of any trials you might be eligible for.

STEP 2: Conduct Research

- **Use reputable online databases.** Some reliable sources of information on clinical trials include:
    - ClinicalTrials.gov: A comprehensive global source of clinical trial information.
    - National Cancer Institute (NCI): Provides trial details specific to cancer research. www.cancer.gov
    - World Health Organization (WHO): The International Clinical Trials Registry Platform (ICTRP) offers a global view of trials for all health conditions. www.who.int/ictrp

- **Check with patient advocacy groups.** Many advocacy groups maintain trial databases and can guide you toward relevant studies while also offering support to help you navigate the clinical trial process. Ask if they can connect you with others who have participated in clinical trials for shared insight and support.

STEP 3: Evaluate Eligibility

- **Review inclusion/exclusion criteria.** Read the eligibility requirements for each trial to see if you qualify. Criteria may include age, gender, type and stage of disease, previous treatment history, and other medical conditions.

- **Confirm with your doctor.** Ask whether your medical history or current treatments might affect your eligibility.

STEP 4: Contact Trial Coordinators

- **Reach out.** Contact the clinical trial coordinators or principal investigators for more information.

- **Ask questions.** Inquire about the trial's purpose, duration, required procedures, potential risks and benefits, and any associated costs.

STEP 5: Understand the Details

- **Review informed consent.** Carefully read the informed consent document, which outlines key details of the trial, including potential risks and benefits.

- **Address concerns.** Ensure all your questions are answered before signing the consent form.

STEP 6: Consider Logistics

- **Assess location.** Consider the location of the trial site in terms of distance, transportation, and feasibility.

- **Weigh time commitment.** Think about how the trial's schedule might affect your daily life and responsibilities.

STEP 7: Assess Financial Aspects

- **Clarify costs and compensation.** Determine what costs are covered by the trial and what expenses you may have to bear. Some trials offer compensation for participation.

- **Verify insurance coverage.** Check whether your health insurance will cover any routine care costs associated with the trial.

STEP 8: Enlist Support

- **Engage family and friends.** Discuss your decision with loved ones for support and practical help, such as transportation or childcare.

- **Seek out support groups.** Join support groups for patients considering or participating in clinical trials.

STEP 9: Enroll in the Trial

- **Complete screening.** If you meet the eligibility criteria and decide to participate, you'll undergo a screening process to confirm your eligibility.

- **Start participation.** Once enrolled, follow the trial protocol as instructed by the research team.

STEP 10: Stay Informed and Engaged

- **Receive updates.** Stay in regular contact with the trial coordinators and attend all scheduled visits.

- **Report concerns.** Immediately report any side effects or issues you experience during the trial.

STEP 11: Monitor and Evaluate

- **Track your health.** Continuously observe how you feel throughout the trial and report any changes or concerns to your care team.

- **Reassess your participation.** Remember, you have the right to withdraw from the trial at any point if you feel uncomfortable or if it's not benefiting you.

Questions to Ask Trial Coordinators

- What is being studied?
- Why do researchers believe this intervention might be effective?
- What are the possible interventions, and how will they be assigned?
- What are the risks, side effects, and benefits compared to current treatments?
- What tests and procedures are involved?
- Who will oversee my medical care during the trial?
- How often will visits be required?
- Will hospitalization be necessary?
- What options are available if I am injured during the study?
- Who will cover the associated costs, and will there be any reimbursements?
- What type of long-term follow-up care is included in this trial?
- If the intervention benefits me, will I continue to receive it after the trial ends?
- How will the trial's results be communicated to me?

Challenges in Qualifying for a Clinical Trial

Here are some factors that can influence whether you qualify for a clinical trial:

- **Specific medical conditions and stage of disease.** Trials often target very specific medical conditions and may require participants to be at a certain stage of the disease. For example, a cancer trial might only be open to patients with a particular type and stage of cancer.

- **Previous treatments.** Some trials require participants to have undergone, or not undergone, certain treatments. For instance, a trial might exclude patients who have previously been treated with a specific drug.

- **Age and gender.** Many trials have age and gender restrictions to focus on the population most likely to benefit from the intervention or to reduce variability.

- **Health status.** Participants often need to meet specific health criteria, such as having a certain level of kidney or liver function or not having other significant medical conditions that could interfere with the study.

- **Lifestyle factors.** Some trials may exclude participants based on lifestyle factors such as smoking, alcohol consumption, or lack of adherence to a healthy diet.

- **Geographic location.** Proximity to the trial site can be a factor, as frequent visits to the study location may be required.

- **Willingness to follow protocol.** Participants must be willing to comply with the trial's procedures and follow-up requirements, which may include frequent visits, taking medications regularly, and undergoing numerous tests.

Given these factors, it's not uncommon for patients to struggle to qualify for clinical trials. Studies published in the *Journal of the National Cancer Institute*[2] show that participation rates for adults with cancer remain low—often just 2 to 8 percent. Despite ongoing efforts to improve access and inclusivity, these numbers have remained largely unchanged over time.

Remember, if you don't qualify for one clinical trial, it doesn't mean that you're out of options. Many patients who are initially ineligible for one study often find success with others. Each trial has unique criteria, so staying diligent and exploring multiple options can increase your chances of finding the right fit.

Armed with the right information and support, you can make choices that reflect your values and comfort level while keeping the door open to possibility, healing, and hope.

PART THREE

GET ORGANZIED

Chapter 12

When and What to Tell Your Employer

"Timing is everything."
—BUCK BRANNAMAN, *The Faraway Horses*

When I was first diagnosed with cancer, I was working diligently as a freelance writer. I had supported myself for decades as a journalist and advertising copywriter, with expertise in health, education, food, finance, and technology. But when I was diagnosed with stage 3 breast cancer, my work life came to a screeching halt. My priorities instantly shifted from landing the next writing gig to scouring the country for the best medical professionals to tackle this cancerous beast head-on. Fortunately, my husband had a reliable job at the time, so luckily, our family still had income. Equally important, his employer offered excellent health benefits.

For that, we are forever grateful.

My husband didn't hesitate to share my diagnosis with his employer, and we were both thankful for the support and flexibility they offered. That kind of workplace understanding made a tough time feel a little more manageable.

Discussing Your Cancer Diagnosis at Work

Sharing your cancer diagnosis at work can be one of the most challenging conversations you'll have during your journey. Deciding when, how, and what to share is influenced by your treatment plan, your comfort level, and the dynamics of your workplace. Fortunately, federal laws like the Americans with Disabilities Act (ADA) and the Family and Medical Leave Act (FMLA) provide critical protections, including the right to reasonable accommodations and job-protected leave. This section will guide you through understanding these laws, timing your disclosure, and navigating these sensitive conversations to ensure you have the support you need.

Understanding Your Rights: ADA and FMLA Protections

The ADA and FMLA provide key protections for employees with cancer. Understanding your rights under these laws can help you feel more confident when approaching your employer:

▶ ADA Protections

The ADA prohibits discrimination based on disability and requires that employers with fifteen or more employees provide reasonable accommodations, such as:

- Modified break schedules
- Flexible or modified work schedules

- Remote work or telecommuting
- Physical workspace modifications
- Job restructuring

However, accommodations are only required if they do not cause "undue hardship" to the employer, meaning they should not impose significant difficulty or expense relative to the employer's resources and size.

▶ FMLA Eligibility

The FMLA provides up to twelve weeks of unpaid, job-protected leave annually, which can be taken intermittently or continuously for treatment or caregiving. FMLA eligibility is available to employees who meet all three of the following criteria:

- Have worked for their employer for at least twelve months
- Have completed at least 1,250 hours of service in the previous twelve months
- Are employed at a location where the company has fifty or more employees within a seventy-five-mile radius

If you're unable to return to work even after using FMLA, other support options may be available.

If You Can't Continue Working During Treatment

If your cancer or treatment prevents you from working for twelve months or more, you may be eligible for Social Security Disability Insurance (SSDI). Some advanced cancers qualify for fast-tracked approval through the Social Security Administration's Compassionate Allowances program. To learn more or start the application process, visit www.ssa.gov or consult a patient advocate who specializes in employment and disability benefits.

Tip: If you live in a state with additional protections (such as California's Paid Family Leave), familiarize yourself with those benefits as well.

If you have questions about how these protections apply to your specific situation, consider consulting a legal advisor or a patient advocate who specializes in employment law. They can provide clarity on your rights and guide you in navigating more complex scenarios.

When to Tell Your Employer

Timing your disclosure is crucial. You may not need to inform your employer about your diagnosis until your treatment plan is established. Once you have details about your treatment schedule and its impact on your work, you can plan the conversation accordingly. For example, if you are having surgery, you might only need to request time off without mentioning your cancer diagnosis. However, if your treatment includes weekly chemotherapy sessions during work hours, it's best to be upfront.

Who to Talk to First: HR or Your Boss?

Once you've decided it's time to disclose your diagnosis, it's equally important to determine whom to approach first. The choice between speaking to HR or your boss depends on your company's culture and structure. Larger organizations typically require HR to be the initial point of contact for handling sensitive matters confidentially and for providing detailed information on policies, benefits, and legal rights. In smaller companies, a direct discussion with your boss might lead to faster, more personalized accommodations.

How to Talk to Your Employer

Before meeting with HR or your boss, consider the following:

- Prepare a list of questions about accommodations and benefits.
- Outline how your treatment may impact your ability to perform daily tasks.
- Share only the details necessary to secure support. Keeping the focus on how your treatment may affect your work will help maintain clarity and protect your privacy.

Keeping Records

Keep track of all discussions with your boss or HR, and save emails related to your diagnosis and requests, as well as your performance reviews. This documentation can be useful if your cancer diagnosis or accommodations are ever held against you. ADA protections continue even after treatment, which is especially important if lingering effects make it difficult to return to your previous responsibilities. Maintaining detailed records will ensure you have documentation to support your case if any issues or questions arise later. This record-keeping can be crucial in protecting your rights.

Managing Self-Employment

Navigating cancer treatment while self-employed presents unique challenges, especially without the safety net of employer-provided benefits. However, there are still valuable resources and support systems to help you manage your health and maintain your livelihood.

- **Health insurance.** Consider purchasing health insurance through the Healthcare Marketplace, where coverage for preexisting conditions, including cancer, is guaranteed. You may qualify for a Special Enrollment Period (SEP) due to life events such as loss of coverage, moving, or a cancer diagnosis. This allows you to obtain insurance soon after your diagnosis. Depending on your income and state, you might also be eligible for subsidies to help lower costs.

- **Financial planning.** Consult with a financial advisor experienced in health crises to help manage your finances. Creating a budget that accounts for both medical expenses and personal living costs can help minimize financial stress during treatment. Local cancer support groups and national organizations like the American Cancer Society (ACS) also offer financial assistance programs for cancer patients.

- **Disability support for the self-employed.** Even as a self-employed individual, you may qualify for Social Security Disability Insurance (SSDI) if your cancer or treatment prevents you from working for twelve months or more. Eligibility depends on your work history and whether you've contributed to Social Security through self-employment taxes. Advanced cancers may qualify for expedited review through the Compassionate Allowances (CAL) program.

Visit www.ssa.gov or speak to a patient advocate for help navigating the application process.

- **Adjusting your workload.** Enlist a trusted colleague or business mentor to help you plan for how to sustain your business without overextending yourself. Consider reducing your hours, taking on less demanding projects, delegating tasks, or hiring temporary help. Setting a realistic schedule and building in time to rest during treatment can help keep your workload manageable. If possible, set clear expectations with clients about project timelines and your availability early on.

- **Accessing support resources.** Local cancer support groups and national organizations, such as the ACS, can connect you with programs specifically designed for self-employed individuals. For financial aid or guidance on managing your business during treatment, contact an ACS representative or visit their website for the latest resources and referrals.

Navigating work and cancer treatment is a deeply personal and often overwhelming challenge, whether you're discussing your diagnosis with your employer or trying to keep your business afloat. Remember to be kind to yourself during this time. Take the time to learn about your rights, reach out for support from HR or trusted professionals, and adapt these strategies in a way that feels right for you.

Every patient's journey is unique, and by equipping yourself with knowledge and preparing thoughtfully, you can create a work environment that supports your well-being, no matter your employment situation. If you ever feel uncertain about your options, consider reaching out to a patient advocate or legal advisor for personalized guidance.

Above all, give yourself permission to focus on what you need—not just to work, but to heal. That may mean leaning on others more than you're used to, stepping back from what doesn't serve you, or simply taking things one day at a time. Your well-being matters more than any task, deadline, or expectation.

Chapter 13

Keep Track of Medical Tests and Records

"A place for everything, and everything in its place."
—NOAH WEBSTER, *The American Spelling Book*

Keeping track of your medical tests and records is a powerful way to take charge of your cancer care. A well-organized record of your medical history, test results, and treatment information not only helps you make informed decisions but also ensures that you and your healthcare team have the most up-to-date information to guide your treatment.

Every cancer diagnosis is accompanied by a series of medical tests and then what feels like a never-ending wait for the results. I remember the anxious days and sleepless nights, waiting for each call or appointment, hoping for some clarity yet dreading what I might hear. Waiting was one of the hardest parts of my journey—a constant reminder that so much was out of my control. But over time, I learned to find moments of calm amid the uncertainty.

Ask When to Expect Your Test Results

Waiting for test results can be one of the most stressful parts of the cancer journey. The uncertainty can feel unbearable, but once you have answers, you can begin to process what's next. With each test, ask when you can expect results. Knowing the timeline can ease some of the anxiety. In the meantime, take gentle care of yourself, and allow others to care for you, too.

Ask How and When You'll Receive Your Test Results

Understanding how and when your results will be delivered can help you prepare both emotionally and practically.

- **Through the patient portal.** Federal regulations require most test results (labs, pathology, imaging reports, etc.) to be released as soon as they're finalized—often before a physician has reviewed them. This means patients may see results, even serious ones, before talking with their doctor. Some hospitals and clinics delay certain "sensitive" results (like biopsy or genetic tests) for 24–72 hours, so a clinician can reach out first. In some systems, patients can opt in to this delay so their doctor has time to reach out before results are posted.

- **Over the phone.** If your test results are going to be delivered by your doctor over the phone, ask for a copy of the report beforehand. That way, you can review it first and create a list of questions to ask during the call.

- **In person.** If your test results are going to be delivered by your doctor during an in-person appointment, be sure to ask for a copy to take home with you. That way, once you're out of the emotionally charged setting, you can take your time to slowly digest the report. If you have any questions that were not discussed at your appointment, jot them down and send them to your doctor via email or your patient portal.

Confirm What You Heard

What doctors say and what patients hear can sometimes differ, especially in high-stress discussions. When reviewing your test results:

- Repeat back what your doctor said, restating what you think you heard. This helps to eliminate potential misunderstandings.
- Find out the implications of your test results.
- Ask whether you need any other testing.

Keep Copies of Important Medical Records

When I was in the midst of treatment, it never occurred to me how important it would become to have the details of my diagnosis and treatment on hand. These records are not only essential during treatment—when you're seeking second and third opinions—but they could also be critical in the future for follow-up care. Although I pride myself on my organizational skills, I'm embarrassed to admit that over twenty years after my diagnosis, I've lost all my cancer treatment records. And I've since learned that medical offices only keep records for a limited time. To receive the best care now and in the future, it's crucial to become the gatekeeper of your own medical history.

The American Cancer Society recommends that you retain the following records:

- Copies of pathology reports from all your biopsies and surgeries
- Copies of imaging test results (e.g., CT or MRI scans), which can usually be stored digitally on a DVD
- If you had surgery, a copy of your operative report(s)
- If you stayed in the hospital, copies of discharge summaries your healthcare provider wrote when you were sent home
- If you received chemotherapy or other drug treatments (such as targeted therapy, immunotherapy, or hormone therapy), a list of the drugs, their doses, and how long you took them
- If you underwent radiation therapy, a copy of your treatment summary
- Contact information for all healthcare providers who treated your cancer

If a new provider requests copies of any of the above information, always keep a copy for yourself.

Maintaining your medical records can feel overwhelming at times, but it's a vital step in becoming your own best advocate. When you have everything documented and accessible, you can focus more on your healing and less on chasing paperwork. Remember, your health is your top priority, and staying organized is a meaningful way to support yourself during this challenging journey.

As you move forward, remember: You don't have to manage everything on your own. Patient navigators and healthcare professionals can be valuable partners in helping you stay organized and informed, giving you greater peace of mind as you navigate your care.

Chapter 14

Manage Your Meds

"An ounce of prevention is worth a pound of cure."
—BENJAMIN FRANKLIN, *Poor Richard's Almanack*

For a newly diagnosed cancer patient, managing medications effectively is a top priority—crucial for both treatment success and quality of life. When I was going through treatment, I found it challenging to stay on top of all my medications, vitamins, and supplements. I felt like I was always taking pills—post-breakfast meds, post-breakfast supplements, meds after lunch, post-lunch supplements, meds after dinner, post-dinner supplements, and meds before bedtime.

On a good day, this may not be a challenge. But if you still have anesthesia in your system, or if you're on pain medication and can't think straight, don't be afraid to enlist the help of a friend or family member to keep your meds on track.

Simplifying Your Pill-Taking Regimen

Whether you're on your own or have help, the following strategies can ease the process of keeping up with your medications:

STEP 1: Create a Medication Schedule

- **List all medications.** Write down all the medications you need to take, including dosage, frequency, and any special instructions. I keep a list of my medications on my phone, so I always have it on hand to share when needed.

- **Use a pill organizer.** A weekly pill organizer with compartments for different times of the day can help prevent missed doses and ensure you're taking the right medication at the right time. Some even come with built-in alarms and removable daily compartments—handy when you're on the go. You can find them at most pharmacies or online.

  Warning: Don't separate narcotics from their original containers. Keep those in the packaging provided by your pharmacy.

STEP 2: Set Reminders

- **Set alarms and alerts.** Use your phone or a medication reminder app to set alerts for when it's time to take your medication.

- **Lean on support.** If reminders aren't working for you or if staying on schedule feels overwhelming, ask a family member or friend to check in regularly to help you stay on track.

STEP 3: Keep a Medication Log

- **Track side effects.** Document any side effects you feel, and tell your healthcare provider. You might need to adjust dosages or change medications.

- **Note changes.** Record any changes in your medication regimen.

STEP 4: Communicate with Your Healthcare Team

- **Ask questions.** Don't hesitate to ask your doctor or pharmacist about anything you don't understand regarding your medications.

- **Provide regular updates.** Keep your healthcare team updated on how you are managing with your medications, especially if you suspect you're having side effects or any difficulties.

STEP 5: Appoint One Doctor to Oversee All Your Prescriptions

- **Ensure that one doctor is reviewing all medications for safety.** When you're on multiple prescriptions—often from different specialists—it's essential that one provider takes responsibility for making sure it's safe to take them together. Without oversight, you risk serious side effects or dangerous interactions, especially with pain medications. Before starting anything new, make sure it's cleared by the doctor managing your medications—or at the very least, by your pharmacist.
- **Keep an up-to-date medication list and share it at every appointment.** This helps prevent errors and ensures that all providers are aware of what you're taking, including prescriptions, over-the-counter drugs, and supplements.

Important Tip: If you're prescribed strong opioids for pain, your doctor may also prescribe NARCAN (naloxone) Nasal Spray. This isn't cause for concern—it's a precautionary measure. NARCAN can reverse the effects of an opioid overdose and is often recommended as part of a responsible pain management plan. If your doctor doesn't mention it, ask whether it would be appropriate to have on hand. *Accidental overdoses can happen,* especially when medications are changed, combined, or misused unintentionally.

Reminder: For your own protection, do not separate narcotics from their original container.

Insights from My Journey

Shortly after my mastectomy, my body was riddled with pain, and my brain was still in a fog from the anesthesia. This led to confusion about my medications. I had a hard time remembering which meds I had taken and when. Looking back, I should have used a daily checklist that listed each medication and its scheduled time. That way, I could have checked them off as I went, leaving nothing to guesswork. In retrospect, it would have been wise to put someone else in charge of managing my meds!

I also suffered from ineffective pain meds—which no one was monitoring—along with mind-altering side effects from meds that should have never been taken together. The result: chronic anxiety, paranoia, and insomnia.

After nearly a week without sleep and proper pain management, my physical and mental well-being spiraled into a place I never want to go again. I tried calling my surgeon who had prescribed the pain meds, but she was on vacation with her family and was unreachable. Out of desperation, I called one of my childhood friends, who lived hours away, and asked her to please come take care of me. She showed up that afternoon.

Luckily, she came from a family of doctors who all chimed in on how to best get me out of my predicament.

Her brother, a psychiatrist, told me that I was experiencing a paradoxical reaction to my pain medication. Instead of relieving pain, the medication heightened my sensitivity to it. Rather than feeling sedated, I experienced mania, anxiety, paranoia, and insomnia. These reactions are relatively rare but can happen depending on how medications are metabolized, preexisting mental health conditions, or interactions with other drugs.

A few days after switching pain medications, I was finally able to think clearly again—and sleep. In hindsight, I should have had access to my surgeon or at least a colleague immediately after surgery.

It's standard practice to designate another physician to cover when the primary doctor is unavailable.

I ultimately hired a psychopharmacologist—a doctor specializing in medications for mental health conditions and their effects on mood, behavior, and cognitive function. I spoke to him regularly to ensure my body could tolerate the mix of the medications I was prescribed. This gave me tremendous peace of mind.

I've since learned that most pharmacies use advanced systems to automatically check for drug interactions, allergies, and other risks. When a new prescription is entered, the system flags any potential issues by comparing it with your current medications. These alerts prompt the pharmacist to review the concern and, if needed, contact your doctor or offer guidance. Still, it's smart to be proactive. If no single doctor is managing all your prescriptions, ask your pharmacist to double-check for interactions. And always say "yes" to the consultation—they're there to help protect you.

Managing medications during cancer treatment can feel overwhelming, especially when you're juggling a complex regimen. However, taking steps to stay organized, being proactive about medication safety, and enlisting support from loved ones or medical professionals can significantly ease the burden. Remember, it's OK to ask for help and to prioritize your health above all else. The journey might be challenging, but with the right tools and support, you can navigate this critical aspect of your treatment with confidence and peace of mind.

Chapter 15

Organize Medical Bills and Insurance Documents

"The shortest way to do many things is
to do only one thing at a time."
—RICHARD CECIL, *The Works of the Rev. Richard Cecil*

When you're going through cancer treatment, the last thing you want to worry about is insurance or medical bills, but unfortunately these are financial realities you'll need to manage. During my own treatment, I made a concerted effort to stay on top of all my health-related expenses, but the constant flood of paperwork and sheer exhaustion from treatment often left me overwhelmed. To help you stay organized and reduce stress, I've outlined some practical tips in this chapter.

Create a Filing System

The best way to prevent getting bogged down in medical paperwork is to create a filing system so that every piece of paper has a "home" that can be easily accessed. This task doesn't need to fall entirely on your shoulders. If your friends and family are wondering how they can help during this challenging time, put their goodwill to work to help you get organized!

▶ Physical Folders

If you have space in a filing cabinet, you can create the file folders that I recommend below and place them there. Otherwise, find a portable, letter-sized file box at an office supply store or online. You will also need letter-sized hanging folders and top-tab, 1/3-cut, letter-sized manila folders. The larger tabs provide extra room for writing.

STEP 1: Create a hanging folder titled **Healthcare Providers**. Then create alphabetized manila file folders labeled with the names of all your doctors, medical facilities, and other healthcare providers. This is where all their correspondence will be filed. Keep a detailed log of all interactions with your healthcare providers, noting the date, the person you spoke with, and key points from your conversations.

STEP 2: Write each of the following categories twice—once on the tab of its hanging folder (you'll need to abbreviate here due to lack of space) and once on the tab of the manila file folder that goes inside the hanging folder. File the folders alphabetically:

- **Bill Follow-Up**

- **Copayments Due**
  Keep track of bills that have been processed by your insurance and show a balance you owe. Once paid, move the bill to the appropriate provider's folder inside the Healthcare Providers hanging folder. Be sure to note the date and method of payment directly on the bill.

- **Denied Claims**

- **FSA Expenses**

- **Insurance Correspondence**

- **Insurance Forms**

- **Insurance Policy**
  Keep a copy of both sides of your insurance card and a copy of your insurance policy here. If you can't find your policy and are employed, ask your human resources department. Your insurance company can also provide a copy.

- **Letters of Medical Necessity**
  Letters from your doctor verifying that services or items are for the diagnosis, treatment, or prevention of a disease or medical condition. These are required by the IRS for certain eligible expenses.

- **Misc Uncovered Medical Expenses**
  Some expenses not covered by insurance may be deductible from federal income taxes, such as mileage to and from medical appointments and prescription drugs. Consult your tax advisor for details.

- **Paid by Insurance**
  Store your insurance company's Explanation of Benefits (EOB) here. Once a claim is paid, attach the EOB to the corresponding claim from the **Sent to Insurance** folder. Place the most recent EOBs on top.

- **Prescriptions**
  File the paper attached to the pharmacy bag. It lists the name, dose, and date of each prescribed drug, the prescribing doctor's name, and often includes instructions for use, side effects, precautions, drug interactions, and your copay.

- **Send to Insurance**
  This is for bills you need to submit for reimbursement. Send them every few weeks to avoid a backlog.

- **Sent to Insurance**
  Keep copies of bills and completed insurance claims. If you don't have a photocopier, you can use your phone to take photos. Then either print them at home or save them as digital files and organize them on your computer.

- **Sick Leave/Family Medical Leave Requests**

- **Travel, Meal, and Lodging Expenses**

▶ Digital Folders

Managing important health-related documents digitally can save time, reduce stress, and ensure everything is accessible when you need it. Here's how to effectively capture, organize, retrieve, secure, and back up your files.

- **Capture**
  - **Scan documents.** Use your phone, scanner, or printer to digitize physical documents such as test results, letters, and prescriptions. ***Tip:*** Look for apps with optical character recognition (OCR) to make scanned text searchable.
  - **Receive digitally.** Request healthcare providers to send letters, test results, and other documents via email or secure patient portals like MyChart.
  - **Take notes.** Use note-taking apps to capture conversations during appointments and attach related files.

- **Organize**
  - **Create folders.** Set up a folder structure in a cloud service like Google Drive, Apple iCloud, or Microsoft OneDrive. Suggested folders include:
    - Test Results
    - Insurance Claims
    - Doctor's Notes
    - Prescriptions
  - **Use file naming conventions.** Name files systematically, e.g., YYYY-MM-DD_TestName_DoctorName.pdf, for easier sorting.
  - **Add tags or labels.** Many cloud services allow tagging or color-coding for further organization (e.g., "Urgent," "Follow-Up").

- **Retrieve**
  - **Use search tools.** Cloud services with robust search features help find documents quickly. OCR-enabled apps allow for searching within scanned documents.
  - **Create email folders.** For documents sent via email, create dedicated folders and use filters to automatically sort incoming messages.

- **Bookmark patient portals.** Keep login details handy for secure portals like MyChart or similar services that store medical information.

- **Secure**
  - **Use two-factor authentication.** Enable this feature for all cloud storage and email accounts to protect sensitive data.
  - **Encrypt files.** Use encryption tools or built-in encryption features on macOS and Windows before uploading highly sensitive documents.
  - **Choose secure apps.** Use apps with built-in encryption for extra protection when scanning or sharing documents.

- **Back Up**
  - **Use cloud storage.** Store files in at least two cloud services for redundancy.
  - **Save to external storage.** Use an encrypted external hard drive or USB flash drive for offline backup.
  - **Enable automatic sync.** Turn on automatic syncing across your devices to ensure files are always up-to-date.

By following these steps, you can efficiently manage your documents while ensuring they remain safe, organized, and easy to access.

Navigate Medical Bills and Insurance with Confidence

▶ Maintain a spreadsheet to track bills and payments.

If possible, keep a spreadsheet to track medical bills, due dates, amounts, payments made, and any outstanding balances. Include columns for insurance payments and out-of-pocket expenses.

▶ Stay on top of deadlines.

Use a calendar to mark important dates, such as bill due dates, follow-up appointments, and deadlines for submitting insurance claims. Set reminders on your phone or computer for upcoming payments or document submissions.

▶ Review EOBs carefully.

Cross-check your medical bills against the EOBs provided by your insurance company to ensure accuracy. Look for discrepancies and contact your insurer for clarification, if needed.

▶ Communicate with your providers and insurers.

Don't hesitate to ask for clarification on any bill or insurance statement you don't understand.

Seek Financial Assistance and Insurance Support

▶ Apply for financial help.

If your finances are limited, ask your medical providers about financial assistance programs that may be available through your hospital, cancer organizations, or your insurer. Consider consulting a financial advisor who specializes in healthcare or cancer-related finances. Another option is to join a support group where you can gather and share information on managing medical bills and insurance.

▶ Research health insurance support.

Several organizations offer helpful resources on health insurance for cancer patients, including:

- American Cancer Society: www.cancer.org/cancer/financial-insurance-matters/understanding-health-insurance.html
- Cancer Support Community: www.cancersupportcommunity.org/article/health-insurance-cancer-patients

▶ Get help with copays, premiums, deductibles, and out-of-pocket costs.

Several foundations and nonprofit organizations that can help are listed below:[1]

- CancerCare: www.cancercare.org/financial_assistance
- Cancer Financial Assistance Coalition (CFAC): www.cancerfac.org
- HealthWell Foundation: www.healthwellfoundation.org
- Blood Cancer United Co-Pay Assistance Program: www.bloodcancerunited.org/financial-assistance/co-pay-assistance-program
- Patient Advocate Foundation Co-Pay Relief: www.patientadvocate.org/connect-with-services/copay-relief
- Patient Access Network (PAN) Foundation: www.panfoundation.org

---

Organizing your medical bills and insurance documents can feel like a daunting task, but creating a system is one of the most practical and empowering ways to support yourself. It helps you stay on top of what's owed, catch mistakes before they snowball, and reduce the financial stress that often accompanies cancer treatment.

More importantly, it's an act of self-advocacy—a way of saying, *I deserve clarity, stability, and peace of mind as I heal.*

And while this part of the journey may feel heavy at times, know that you can lean on others when the weight becomes too much. A little help with your paperwork isn't just practical—it's a quiet reminder that you're not in this alone.

PART FOUR

BUILD RESILIENCE FOR THE ROAD AHEAD

Chapter 16

How Nutrition Can Help You Heal

"A well-regulated diet is a medicine in itself."
—LUCIUS ANNAEUS SENECA, *Moral Letters to Lucilius*

Why Nutrition Matters

During my first visit to an oncologist, I asked whether I should change my diet.

He replied, "I wouldn't change a thing. You've got enough changes to deal with—you don't need to change your diet, too."

While I understood his intent, I knew in that moment he wasn't the right doctor for me. I couldn't ignore what I deeply believed: Nutrition isn't optional—it's central to healing.

According to a study published by Cambridge University Press, patients with cancer are among the most malnourished of all patient groups.[1] A comprehensive review of cancer-related malnutrition highlights that systemic inflammation, often present in cancer, increases the body's metabolic needs while depressing appetite and accelerating muscle protein breakdown.

This can lead to cachexia—a severe wasting syndrome marked by significant weight and muscle loss—which affects up to 80 percent of cancer patients at certain stages of their illness.[2]

The same study also emphasizes that people with cancer often face physiological challenges such as malabsorption, vomiting, and diarrhea, all of which contribute to their high risk of malnutrition. These symptoms, combined with the side effects from chemotherapy and radiation, can further worsen nutritional deficiencies.[3]

The Prevalence of Malnutrition in Oncology (PreMiO) study—conducted on 1,952 cancer patients and published in *Oncotarget*—found that malnutrition was prevalent even at the first medical oncology visit, highlighting the need for early nutritional intervention.[4] These findings underscore the critical importance of nutritional assessment and support for cancer patients to improve their treatment outcomes and quality of life.

Food as a Healing Partner

Although cancer treatment can take a toll on your body, you can greatly reduce its effects by making mindful choices about what you consume. The nutritional lessons I learned during my cancer treatment not only helped boost my immune system, combat fatigue, and ward off nasty side effects—they also gave me the chance to lay a new nutritional foundation for my mind and body, both during and after treatment.

To strengthen my immune system, I ultimately added a nutrition-focused integrative oncologist from Chicago to my medical team. I believe that working with Dr. Keith Block—renowned for blending conventional medicine with scientifically supported complementary therapies—played a key role in my healing. I quickly realized that if I wanted the best possible chance at healing, I needed to completely rethink my relationship with food.

Prior to my diagnosis, I was a long-time lover of rich, cancer-promoting foods high in fat, dairy, and sugar—all of which fuel inflammation. In the eighties and early nineties, I worked as a food writer for dozens of companies and commodity boards, including (ironically) the Beef Industry Council. I had always loved eating beef. But after my diagnosis, I learned that conventionally raised beef can promote inflammation in the body, and chronic inflammation is known to contribute to the development and progression of cancer. Beef can also contain saturated fat, carcinogenic compounds, growth hormones, and antibiotics.

Fortunately, just a few months after my diagnosis, a flyer promoting a class series called *Creative Culinary Solutions for Prevention & Healing* arrived in the mail. I enrolled immediately and invited a friend to join me on my quest to learn how to create immune-boosting meals that would nourish me—and still appeal to my family's palate.

Finding Nourishment in the Unexpected

After a scenic forty-five-minute drive through West Marin, my friend and I arrived at a gorgeous private home with an exhibition kitchen. We were greeted by our spirited instructor, Rebecca Katz, whose recipes featured fresh, seasonal, and organic ingredients.

I'll never forget the day Rebecca rolled out her "Cashmere Sweater Soup Collection." Each luscious spoonful wrapped around our tongues like liquid velvet, prompting a chorus of pleasure-filled moans. Yet I couldn't help but wonder, "*This* will help me heal?" and "How could these creamy concoctions contain no dairy?" The answers began to unfold at this sacred place, where I could go for three savory hours every Thursday after chemo to learn, laugh, and take a break from cancer.

A few weeks after finishing Rebecca's first series of cooking classes, I faced the surgery I dreaded most: a bilateral mastectomy.

While the operation went as well as expected, it took weeks for my mind and body to recover from the initial shock. Just ten days after this highly invasive procedure, I hosted my first cooking class, with Rebecca taking center stage. The attendees—generous friends and family members—came eager to learn how to prepare meals that would support my healing journey.

Rebecca went on to write one of Amazon's best-selling cancer cookbooks, titled *The Cancer-Fighting Kitchen: Nourishing Big-Flavor Recipes for Cancer Treatment and Recovery*. It's filled with recipes that nourish not just the immune system, but the soul. My favorite? Magic Mineral Broth. This energizing elixir is high in potassium and numerous trace minerals that are often depleted by cancer therapy.

Your Nutritional Journey: Where to Begin

Below are some suggestions on how nutrition can support your health and well-being during treatment. While much of this information stems from what I learned during my own cancer journey, I've also included insights I wish I'd known at the time. Every patient's needs are unique, shaped by their specific type of cancer and treatment plan. These suggestions are here to guide and support you, but they aren't one-size-fits-all. The best choices are the ones you make in partnership with your care team and in alignment with your body's unique needs.

All the information in this section has been verified by Natalie Ledesma, MS, RDN, CSO, CLT. With over twenty-five years of experience as a registered dietitian nutritionist, Natalie is a seasoned practitioner. A board-certified specialist in oncology nutrition, she serves as the clinical nutrition specialist at Smith Integrative Oncology in San Francisco and is the founding dietitian for the nutrition program at the University of California, San Francisco Helen Diller Family Comprehensive Cancer Center.

Partner with a Cancer Nutrition Specialist

Most cancer facilities have someone on staff who can offer nutritional support. If possible, seek out a CSO, a certified specialist in oncology nutrition. CSOs are registered dietitian nutritionists (RDNs) who have passed a specialized certification exam (which must be retaken every five years) and have completed over two thousand hours working with oncology patients. If your facility doesn't have a CSO, see if you can get a referral from your oncologist, a member of your medical support team, or even a fellow cancer patient.

Keep Your Care Team in the Loop About Supplements

If you're taking any vitamins, minerals, or herbal supplements, be sure to inform your doctor, nurse, and dietitian. It's important they understand everything you're using so they can make sure it all works safely with your treatment plan. Some supplements can be beneficial, but others might interfere with your treatment or make it less effective.

Create a Culinary Support System

During my treatment, I was amazed by how many friends and family members wanted to help—they just needed to know how.

Creating a simple support system around food gave them a meaningful way to show up for me, and it helped me stay nourished when I needed it most.

If your loved ones are offering to help, consider inviting them to support you with meals. Many people are relieved to be given something tangible and helpful to do. While the online scheduling tools available today weren't around when I was going through treatment, they can be a lifesaver when it comes to coordinating support. You'll find a few easy-to-use options in Chapter 3: Enlist the Help of Loved Ones.

For nourishing, great-tasting recipes—soups, meals, snacks, and soothing drinks—I recommend *The Cancer-Fighting Kitchen* by Rebecca Katz and *The Cancer Diet Cookbook* by Dionne Detraz.

Choose Organic When You Can

Organic foods often have more protective phytochemicals, such as antioxidants, than their conventionally grown counterparts. In addition, eating organic reduces the amount of chemicals in your diet, namely pesticides. If availability or cost is a barrier, you might want to avoid the fruits and vegetables with the highest pesticide residues. The Environmental Working Group (EWG) publishes annual "Dirty Dozen" and "Clean Fifteen" lists, which detail the produce with the highest and lowest pesticide levels. You can find this information on their website: www.ewg.org/foodnews.

What to Limit—and Why

The following foods are best minimized during treatment, as they can contribute to inflammation, blood sugar spikes, or impaired healing:

- Foods made with refined sugars, such as cakes, cookies, sweetened cereals, pastries, sodas, fruit drinks, and sweetened tea or coffee
- Foods made with refined or processed grains or flour, such as white bread and white pasta
- Alcohol
- Inflammatory foods such as red meat and dairy

  Note: If you eat red meat, choose high-quality, grass-fed, organic sources. For dairy, select organic options—ideally unsweetened and fermented such as yogurt or kefir.
- Processed meats, such as hot dogs and cold cuts
- Excess coffee

Smart, Nourishing Options to Keep on Hand

When your energy is low or your appetite isn't strong, having simple, nourishing options within reach can make a big difference. Here are a few foods and beverages that are gentle, supportive, and easy to keep nearby.

- Thermos-friendly options: broth, green tea, ginger tea, herbal tea, and unsweetened flavored water (e.g., cucumber, lemon, or mint)
- Sparkling water (which can help settle your stomach)
- Green vegetable juices
- Most nuts and seeds: walnuts, almonds, pistachios, hazelnuts, Brazil nuts, chia seeds, flax seeds, hemp hearts, and pumpkin seeds
- Hard-boiled eggs (preferably organic and pasture-raised)
- Soup
- Smoothies

Smoothie Tips: Use whole fruits with their skin when possible to retain fiber, which helps regulate blood sugar and supports digestion. Limit added sugars like honey or syrup. Balance with vegetables such as spinach, kale, or carrots for added nutrients and fiber. For staying power, include a source of protein—such as Greek yogurt or protein powder—and healthy fats like avocado, nut butters (almond, peanut, or cashew), or seeds. Choose low-glycemic fruits like berries, apples, and pears, which are gentler on blood sugar than high-glycemic options like bananas or mangoes. Watch portion sizes to avoid excess sugar.

When You're Not Hungry (But Need to Eat)

- Be sure to have some food in your stomach. You are more likely to feel nauseous if your stomach is empty.
- If your appetite is diminished or your digestion is compromised, consider eating several small meals throughout the day instead of three main ones.
- If food tastes metallic, it could indicate a zinc deficiency. Consider requesting a zinc test from your healthcare practitioner. You may need to increase your protein intake or add a zinc supplement. To help avoid the metallic taste, try using chopsticks or bamboo utensils instead of metal ones.
- If taste is blunted, try the FASS technique (Fat, Acid, Salt, Sweet) to enhance the flavor of your food. Use natural sweeteners like honey or pure maple syrup.
- If your mouth is dry, eat or drink something tart before meals to stimulate saliva production, which can improve how things taste.

- If you're struggling to find foods that appeal to you or sit well in your stomach, these options are gentle, nourishing, and easy to digest:
    - Bone broth
    - Smoothies with protein powder
    - Soups
    - Avocado
    - Coconut and coconut-based products
    - Chia pudding

      To make chia pudding, stir three tablespoons of chia seeds into one cup of unsweetened plant-based milk (such as almond, oat, or coconut), then refrigerate for at least four hours or overnight until it thickens to a pudding-like consistency.

Before Surgery: Build a Healing Foundation

What you eat in the days or weeks leading up to surgery can have a significant impact on your ability to heal, your immune response, and even your risk of complications. Focus on nutrient-dense, anti-inflammatory foods that support tissue repair, stabilize blood sugar, and strengthen your immune system.

▶ 1. Protein-Rich Foods

Protein is essential for wound healing and maintaining muscle mass. Include high-quality sources such as:

- Lean poultry, fish, and eggs
- Plant-based options like tofu, lentils, and chickpeas. Tofu and other whole soy foods are generally safe in moderation, and some studies suggest they may even offer protective

benefits. If you've been diagnosed with a hormone-sensitive cancer, it's a good idea to check with your doctor or dietitian to see what's best for you.
- Greek yogurt or kefir

▶ 2. Anti-Inflammatory Fruits and Vegetables

Aim for a colorful plate. These foods are rich in vitamins, antioxidants, and fiber:

- Berries, oranges, spinach, kale, broccoli, and bell peppers
- Apples (a low glycemic fruit) and pears, which are great for fiber and easy to digest

▶ 3. Whole Grains

Choose complex carbs to provide lasting energy and stabilize blood sugar:

- Quinoa, brown rice, oats, and barley
- Limit refined carbs like white bread or sugary cereals

▶ 4. Healthy Fats

Omega-3 fatty acids may help reduce inflammation and promote healing:

- Fatty fish (like salmon)
- Flaxseeds and walnuts
- Olive oil and avocados

▶ 5. Hydration

Staying well-hydrated improves circulation, supports detoxification, and aids digestion:

- Drink plenty of water, herbal teas, and broths
- Minimize caffeine and avoid alcohol

Tip: Discontinue most dietary supplements at least seven days before surgery, as many—such as curcumin, CoQ10, and medicinal mushrooms—may have blood-thinning effects. Always consult your physician for guidance. In the days leading up to surgery, also avoid high-sodium, ultra-processed foods and added sugars, which can increase inflammation and interfere with healing.

After Surgery: Fuel Your Recovery

Your body will be in active repair mode after surgery, so postoperative nutrition is just as important—if not more so—than what you eat before the procedure. The right foods can support tissue regeneration, reduce inflammation, restore energy, and prevent complications like constipation or infection.

▶ 1. Prioritize Easy-to-Digest Proteins

Post-surgery, your body needs extra protein to rebuild tissue and fight infection. Start with gentler options if your appetite is low.

- Eat soft scrambled eggs or well-cooked lentils.
- Drink protein smoothies, bone broth, or collagen-rich soups.
- Choose Greek yogurt or cottage cheese.

▶ 2. Consume Anti-Inflammatory Fruits and Vegetables

These provide essential vitamins (like A and C) and fiber:

- Start with cooked vegetables, which are easier to digest, like carrots, squash, and spinach.

- Choose soft fruits, which are gentle on digestion, like bananas, applesauce, and blueberries.
- Reintroduce raw produce gradually, as your body tolerates it.

▶ 3. Choose Healthy Complex Carbs for Fiber and Sustained Energy

Surgery and pain medications often slow digestion. To support digestion and maintain energy:

- Eat sweet potatoes, pumpkin, or winter squash.
- Try oatmeal, quinoa, brown rice, or whole grain toast.
- Add chia or flaxseeds to smoothies or oatmeal for extra fiber.

▶ 4. Include Healthy Fats for Healing

To support cellular repair and absorb fat-soluble vitamins (A, D, E, K):

- Add avocados, olive oil, nuts, seeds, and fatty fish to your diet.
- Avoid greasy, fried foods, which can slow recovery.

▶ 5. Stay Well Hydrated

After surgery, dehydration can increase fatigue, constipation, and even confusion:

- Sip water regularly throughout the day.
- Incorporate herbal teas, diluted juices, and electrolyte broths into your daily routine.

▶ 6. Support Gut Health with Prebiotics, Probiotics, and Polyphenols

Antibiotics and anesthesia can disrupt your gut microbiome. To restore balance:

- Eat prebiotic-rich foods like berries, garlic, leeks, mushrooms, jicama, artichokes, ground flax seed, and dandelion greens.
- Include probiotic options, such as sauerkraut, kimchi, kombucha, miso, apple cider vinegar, unsweetened kefir, or unsweetened yogurt. Consider a probiotic supplement if recommended by your doctor.
- Enjoy polyphenol-rich foods like berries, green tea, matcha, pomegranates, cherries, coffee, black olives, capers, and artichokes.

▶ 7. Take Supplements to Support Surgical Healing

During recovery, your body may benefit from added nutritional support. The following supplements are commonly used to promote healing—just be sure to consult your doctor first:

- Vitamin A
- Vitamin C
- Zinc

Eating Well to Ease Chemo Brain

While there's no magic food that can make chemo brain disappear, certain dietary choices may help support brain function, boost energy, and improve mental clarity during treatment. These include:

- Water
- Walnuts
- Fatty fish like salmon, herring, sardines, and mackerel
- Turmeric
- Blueberries
- Dark, leafy greens like spinach

- Avocados
- Eggs
- Celery
- Rosemary
- Olive oil

As you move through your treatment journey, remember that food is one of the most powerful tools to support your body's healing. Thoughtful, informed choices about what you eat and drink can help ease side effects, strengthen your immune system, and lay a foundation for lasting wellness.

By choosing nourishing, healing foods, you're not only fueling your recovery, you're actively participating in your own care. Embracing nutrition is an act of self-respect, resilience, and hope. For me, it became a daily reminder that even in the midst of cancer, I could nourish not just my body—but my spirit, too.

Chapter 17

Where to Find Emotional Support

"We are each of us angels with only one wing;
and we can only fly by embracing one another."
—LUCIANO DE CRESCENZO, *Così parlò Bellavista*
(Thus Spoke Bellavista)

By day, I was surrounded by family and friends, but in the middle of the night, I had never felt so alone. I felt that my body had betrayed me and was now forcing me to embark on a journey that I didn't want to take. But the people I met along the way turned out to be just the remedy I needed. They helped ease my loneliness—and became an essential part of my healing. I just needed time to let them in.

When I was first diagnosed, the thought of going to a cancer support group was out of the question. I could barely process my own pain—taking on anyone else's felt unimaginable. But after months of trying to tough it out alone, the weight of emotional isolation finally pushed me to show up.

To my surprise, I found comfort in realizing how much we had in common. We also shared information about the local medical community that ultimately changed the course of my medical care. For that, I will be forever grateful. We were truly kindred spirits and lucky to have found one another.

I didn't know it at the time, but walking into that room was one of the most important choices I made during treatment. Still, getting there wasn't easy.

Is a Support Group Right for You?

If you're on the fence, you're not alone. Opening up to strangers isn't easy. Yet many people turn to support groups to connect with others who truly understand what they're going through and to feel less alone in the process. These groups can ease anxiety and stress while offering practical advice, encouragement, and a sense of hope.

Most cancer support groups do not charge a fee to participate. These groups are often sponsored by hospitals, cancer organizations, and community groups, which typically provide their services for free. However, some private or specialized support groups might charge a fee, so it's always a good idea to check with the specific group you are interested in joining. Many organizations aim to make support accessible to all who need it, regardless of their financial situation.

The Healing Power of Connection

Research shows just how powerful social connection can be, especially for people facing serious health challenges like cancer.

One large review of 148 studies involving more than three hundred thousand people found that individuals with strong social relationships had a 50 percent greater chance of survival.[1] Another major review of 87 studies found that cancer patients who felt well-supported had a 15–25 percent lower risk of dying from the disease. Researchers believe this benefit comes not only from emotional support but also from the practical help that makes it easier to manage treatment and stay on top of self-care.[2]

The Life After Breast Cancer Epidemiology (LACE) study echoed these findings, showing that women with larger social networks had lower mortality rates. These studies make it clear: Support isn't just comforting. It can be lifesaving.[3]

Trying a Support Group: What to Expect

Trying a support group for the first time can feel awkward, and it's natural to need time to adjust. But if you're curious, I encourage you to give it a few tries before deciding whether it's right for you. If there are multiple options in your area—or online—visit a few and notice which one feels most comfortable. With a little patience and openness, you may find a group that offers the kind of support you didn't know you needed.

Questions to Ask Before Joining a Support Group[4]

- How large is the group?
- Who attends (survivors, family members, types of cancer, age range)?
- How long are the meetings?
- How often does the group meet?
- How long has the group been together?
- Who leads the meetings—a professional or a survivor?
- What is the format of the meetings?

- Is the main purpose to share feelings, or do people also offer tips to solve common problems?
- If I go, can I just sit and listen?

Types of Support Groups

- **In-person support groups.** General cancer support groups welcome patients with any type of cancer, offering a broad sense of community. Type-specific groups, such as those for breast or prostate cancer, provide more tailored discussions and resources.

- **Online support groups.** Available anytime, online groups let you connect through forums, chats, webinars, and social media—day or night, from the comfort of home. Many are moderated by professionals or hosted by trusted organizations, helping you feel safe and supported. Be sure to choose a group that's monitored, and always double-check any medical advice with your doctor.

- **Telephone support groups.** These groups function like conference calls. They are often free or low-cost and provide a simple way to connect from anywhere.

- **Peer-to-peer support.** Peer support is deeply personal, connecting you one-on-one with someone who has gone through a similar experience. Formats include:
    - Mentorship programs (in person, video, phone, email, or online chat)
    - Support hotlines
    - Face-to-face meetings
    - Online forums and communities

Where to Find a Local In-Person Support Group

Local support may be closer than you think:

- Ask your hospital or cancer center about their support programs.
- Talk to a social worker or your oncologist for referrals.
- Connect with other patients who may know of local groups.

Online Communities and Professional Support Services

The organizations below offer moderated forums, professional guidance, and emotional support through online platforms. Some also offer in-person services or additional resources for caregivers.

- **Cancer Survivors Network (CSN)**
  https://csn.cancer.org
  An online forum hosted by the American Cancer Society. A safe space where members share personal stories, ask questions, and support one another on topics like survivorship, recovery, and treatment effects. Moderated to foster respect and accuracy.

- **CancerCare**
  www.cancercare.org/support_groups
  A national nonprofit that provides free online support groups moderated by professional oncology social workers. Groups use 24/7 message boards so participants can post at

their own pace. CancerCare also offers individual counseling, education programs, and limited financial help.

- **Cancer Support Community**
  www.cancersupportcommunity.org
  A global organization providing free online and in-person services that support mind-body wellness. Resources include support groups, individual counseling, nutrition and fitness programs, and workshops on emotional coping and self-care.

- **Smart Patients**
  www.smartpatients.com
  A moderated online community for patients and caregivers. Conversations are led by people with lived experience, while health professionals and researchers help ensure information is accurate. Topics include treatment, side effects, and emotional support.

- **Inspire**
  www.inspire.com
  A health-centered social platform connecting people through disease-specific communities. Built in partnership with advocacy organizations, it offers privacy-focused forums for sharing experiences, asking questions, and offering mutual encouragement.

Remote Peer Support

Some organizations offer "buddy" programs—personalized peer support with trained volunteers who have been through a similar diagnosis and treatment.

- **American Cancer Society CARES (Community Access to Resources, Education, and Support)**
  www.cancer.org/support-programs-and-services/acs-cares.html
  The ACS CARES mobile app is a free support tool for people with cancer and their loved ones, offering 24/7 access to expert guidance, personalized information, and connections to trained volunteers with similar experiences. The app also offers in-person support at select clinics and is available in Spanish when your phone is set to that language.

- **Imerman Angels**
  www.imermanangels.org
  A nonprofit that connects cancer patients, survivors, and caregivers with trained volunteer mentors—called "Mentor Angels"—who have lived through a similar diagnosis and treatment. Support is available via phone, video, or email.

- **Friend for Life Cancer Support Network**
  www.friend4life.org
  A community-based organization that pairs newly diagnosed patients or their loved ones with volunteers who've faced similar cancer experiences, offering support throughout treatment and recovery.

- **Colorectal Cancer Alliance Buddy Program**
  https://colorectalcancer.org/resources-support/community-support/buddy-program

A peer support program for individuals with colorectal cancer. Participants are matched with survivors who offer encouragement and insights into treatment, side effects, and recovery.

- **GO2 for Lung Cancer Phone Buddy Program**
  https://go2.org/resources-and-support/emotional-support/phone-buddy
  A support program that pairs lung cancer patients and caregivers with trained volunteers for one-on-one phone conversations that offer guidance and understanding.

- **4th Angel Mentoring Program**
  https://4thangel.ccf.org
  A Cleveland Clinic initiative that offers free peer mentoring for cancer patients and caregivers. Trained survivors connect via phone, email, or online chat to provide personalized, one-on-one support.

Other Forms of Local Support

While online support can be incredibly helpful, there's something especially comforting about connecting with someone face-to-face. These connections can offer not just emotional grounding, but also referrals and resources you might not find on your own.

- **Therapists.** Licensed mental health professionals who specialize in helping people navigate serious illness. They provide a safe space to process emotions, reduce anxiety, and build emotional resilience. Ask your care team for a referral.

- **Oncology social workers.** Licensed professionals based in most hospitals and cancer centers. They provide emotional support, help patients and families navigate the treatment process, and maintain up-to-date referrals to local services and support groups.

- **Spiritual care providers.** Whether chaplains, clergy, or other spiritual advisors, they can offer emotional guidance and help connect you to additional community resources.

Emotional support can be just as vital to your healing as the treatment itself. Whether you join a group, connect with a mentor, or find comfort online, the right kind of support can help lighten your emotional load. Take time to explore what feels right, and give yourself permission to lean on others. You deserve to feel seen, understood, and supported.

Chapter 18

How Gratitude Can Improve Your Recovery

"Gratitude is an emotion that grounds us
and is a great way to balance out the negative
mindset that uncertainty engenders."
—DR. GUY WINCH, *Harvard Business Review*

When I was newly diagnosed, the first person I called was my sister. After we shared a good cry, she said something that has stayed with me ever since: "If you have cancer, I have cancer." Those words filled me with profound love and gratitude, feelings that remain with me to this day.

A cancer diagnosis brings with it an unsettling sense of uncertainty. None of us ever really knows what tomorrow will bring, but if you're a cancer patient, that uncertainty is especially hard to ignore. Even just waiting for test results can be enough to push your anxiety meter into the red zone.

One way to counter that uncertainty is to focus on the people and things you *can* rely on. Whether it's friends and family, community support, or the care and dedication of your healthcare team, taking a moment to appreciate what you have can be a simple yet powerful act of kindness—toward yourself and others. It can ease anxiety and bring a sense of calm to challenging times.

What Is Gratitude?

Gratitude is more than a polite thank-you or a fleeting feeling—it's a way of seeing the world through a lens of grace. At its heart, gratitude is a spiritual practice, an acknowledgment that life holds goodness, even in the midst of difficulty. It invites us to pause and recognize the blessings—big and small—that often come from outside ourselves: the love of others, the beauty of nature, small acts of kindness, or a sense of something greater than ourselves.

The *Oxford English Dictionary* defines gratitude as "the quality or condition of being thankful; the appreciation of and inclination to return kindness." Practicing gratitude helps us shift our focus to what is present and life-affirming, instead of what is missing or uncertain.

Living with gratitude lays the foundation for a more hopeful, open-hearted life. This doesn't mean denying the pain or pretending everything is fine. It means choosing not to let suffering eclipse the goodness that still exists.

Gratitude in Spiritual Traditions

In Judaism, the first words of the morning prayer can be translated as, "I thank you." The Hebrew term for gratitude is *hakarat hatov*, which means, literally, "recognizing the good." Gratitude is also a vital part of Christianity; before Jesus has his last meal with his disciples, he gives thanks. Gratitude is deeply rooted in

Islam, too. The Quran lists blessings for which people should be grateful—like the sun, moon, clouds, rain, plants, and oceans—and then asks, "How can a sensible person be anything but thankful to God?"

Other traditions also stress the importance of thankfulness. Hindu festivals celebrate blessings and offer thanks for them. In Buddhism, gratitude helps develop the virtue of patience. People with a strong sense of gratitude are more likely to be able to delay gratification, passing on a small reward now in favor of a greater reward later. This ties in with the Buddhist belief that gratitude is the antidote to greed. Gratitude reminds us that what we have is enough.

How Gratitude Supports Healing

According to Dr. Robert Emmons, professor of psychology at UC Davis and a pioneer in the science of gratitude, "The practice of gratitude can have dramatic and lasting effects in a person's life."

His research has shown that gratitude can bring the following benefits:[1]

- **Lower blood pressure.** Research demonstrates that gratitude can significantly reduce blood pressure. In a study led by Dr. Emmons, participants who kept gratitude journals experienced measurable drops in blood pressure over time. These findings align with a growing body of evidence suggesting that gratitude practices can have tangible, positive effects on cardiovascular health.

- **Stronger immune function.** The relationship between gratitude and improved immune function can be partially explained by its effects on cortisol levels. Cortisol is a hormone released in response to stress, and chronic high levels of cortisol can suppress the immune system, leading to increased inflammation and a higher risk of illness. Gratitude lowers stress hormones like cortisol, which can otherwise weaken the immune system and increase inflammation.

- **Better sleep.** Studies by Dr. Emmons and others show that gratitude can lead to better sleep by shifting your focus away from worry and toward what's good in your life. This positive impact on sleep is linked to the way gratitude fosters a more optimistic and peaceful state of mind. People who regularly express gratitude tend to focus on positive experiences and relationships, reducing the likelihood of being consumed by worries or negative thoughts as they prepare for sleep. Those who practice gratitude tend to drift off more easily, sleep more soundly, and wake up feeling more restored.

- **Less depression and anxiety.** Gratitude helps shift focus from fear and negativity to hope and connection. That shift can reduce the risk of depression and anxiety, promote emotional resilience, and ease feelings of hopelessness by deepening social bonds and helping people find meaning in difficult times.

- **More happiness and emotional well-being.** Gratitude increases the production of dopamine and serotonin—two key neurotransmitters that help regulate mood. Dopamine fuels motivation and reward; serotonin promotes calm and emotional steadiness. Together, these brain chemicals help you feel more balanced, connected, and resilient.[2]

How to Cultivate Gratitude

Gratitude can be practiced anytime, anywhere. Here are a few ways to bring more of it into your daily life.

- **Keep a gratitude journal.** Each day, write down three specific things you're grateful for. Try to journal at the same time each day to create a habit. Studies show journaling before bed can improve your sleep.

- **Write thank-you notes.** Once a month, send a note of thanks to someone who's made a difference in your life. It doesn't have to be fancy—just heartfelt. One study found that people in counseling who wrote gratitude letters felt better, faster.

- **Thank someone mentally.** No time to write? Just pause and think of someone who's shown you kindness. Emmons's research shows that even silently feeling gratitude can lift your mood and enhance your overall well-being.

- **Schedule gratitude visits.** Make time to visit people who've supported you. Your presence will mean the world to them, and you'll likely feel uplifted in return.

- **Take gratitude walks.** While walking, reflect on what you're grateful for. Choose a tree or special landmark as your "gratitude touchpoint." Each time you pass it, acknowledge its beauty and presence. Chances are, you'll return feeling lighter and more at peace.

- **Practice gratitude at meals.** Start mealtime with a moment of gratitude. If you're with others, go around the table and share something each person is grateful for. If you're alone, take a quiet moment before your first bite.

- **Use visual reminders.** Choose an object in your surroundings that brings up a happy memory. In difficult moments, focus on that object and let it be a reminder of your gratitude.

- **Give yourself a compliment.** Try standing in front of a mirror and naming three things you appreciate about yourself. Maybe it's your loyalty, creativity, or courage. Say them out loud . . . then give yourself a moment to let the words sink in.

- **Pray.** If you're religious, prayer can be a powerful way to express gratitude and reflect on life's blessings. Over time, prayer can foster peace, purpose, and a sense of connection.

Gratitude may begin as a feeling, but with practice, it becomes a way of living. Whether through journaling, appreciating others, or simply noticing the good around you, a regular gratitude practice can help you feel calmer, stronger, and more hopeful. Start small. Stay consistent. And notice how this simple shift brings more light to your healing journey.

PART FIVE

BOOST YOUR MIND, BODY, AND SPIRIT

Chapter 19

Meditation

> "Nowhere can man find a quieter or more untroubled retreat than in his own soul."
> —MARCUS AURELIUS, *Meditations*

Shortly after my diagnosis, I landed an appointment with UCSF's leading breast cancer oncologist for a second opinion. I had already met with a specialist at Stanford, but the aggressive treatment plan he proposed felt too extreme at the time.

On the way to that pivotal consultation—one that could reshape the course of my treatment—I noticed a small chapel tucked off the corridor. Drawn by something I couldn't quite name, I stepped inside. The noise of the hospital fell away. Sitting quietly, I turned my attention to my breath and grounded myself in the present moment, carving out a pocket of calm to gently reflect on the weighty decisions ahead.

For the first time in weeks, I felt a deep sense of peace—a powerful reminder that tending to my mental and emotional well-being was just as essential as choosing the right medical team and treatment.

People have turned to meditation for thousands of years to find calm, deepen self-awareness, and reconnect with something greater than themselves. At its heart, meditation is about gently focusing your attention—often on the breath, a word, or a feeling—to steady the mind and release emotional tension.

Meditation cultivates mindfulness—the ability to be fully present in the moment. This gentle awareness allows you to observe your thoughts and emotions without getting swept up in them. Over time, meditation has branched into many styles, like mindfulness meditation, transcendental meditation, and guided imagery. Each one offers something different, but they all help bring clarity to the mind and steadiness to the heart.

These styles grew out of ancient traditions. Meditation has deep roots in Eastern traditions like Hinduism, Buddhism, and Taoism, where it was used as a path to spiritual awakening and inner wisdom. In these practices, meditation helped people move beyond mental distractions, open their hearts, and connect with the divine.

Over time, meditation spread to the West—first through spiritual communities, then into hospitals and health centers. Today, people all over the world turn to meditation not just for spiritual growth, but for practical support with stress, anxiety, and emotional health.

In today's healthcare settings—especially cancer care—meditation is often used as a helpful complement to treatment. By promoting relaxation and mental clarity, meditation can ease stress, lessen anxiety, and even help with pain, giving patients more peace and resilience as they move through treatment.

In the midst of a cancer diagnosis, meditation can provide a sanctuary of calm and clarity. It helps you turn inward, tap into your inner strength, and find a bit of steadiness when everything feels out of control. When practiced regularly, meditation becomes a constant companion, nurturing a deep sense of calm and supporting recovery during this challenging time.

How Meditation Supports Cancer Care

▶ Stress Relief

Stress is one of the most common challenges during cancer treatment. Meditation offers a simple yet powerful way to manage it. By helping you stay grounded in the present moment, meditation interrupts the cycle of worry and fear about what lies ahead. This shift can lower cortisol levels—the body's main stress hormone—which often spike during cancer treatment. As cortisol drops, the body relaxes, relieving tension, headaches, and fatigue. With regular practice, meditation can bring a deeper sense of calm and help you feel steadier through the ups and downs of treatment.[1]

▶ Pain Management

Pain is a part of the journey for many people going through cancer. Meditation offers a gentle, drug-free way to ease that pain. Practices like mindfulness and guided imagery can help shift your focus away from discomfort and toward more neutral or calming sensations.

Meditation also stimulates the release of endorphins—your body's natural painkillers. Additionally, meditation changes how the brain interprets pain signals, making the pain feel less intense. Over time, adding meditation to your routine may help reduce your need for medication and make pain easier to manage.[2]

▶ Immune Support

Your immune system plays a vital role in your ability to fight cancer, and research suggests that meditation can help strengthen it.

Stress and anxiety can weaken your immune response, making it harder for your body to combat illness. By reducing stress, meditation supports your immune system, increasing the activity of natural killer cells and other immune defenders that work to protect you.

Studies show that regular meditation practice can improve immune markers, including higher antibody levels and a stronger cellular response. This boost is especially important as you recover from treatments like chemotherapy and radiation.[3]

▶ Emotional Balance

Anxiety and depression are common after a cancer diagnosis, and meditation can be a powerful tool for managing both. Mindfulness meditation, in particular, helps break the cycle of negative thinking that fuels fear and despair. By anchoring your attention in the present and observing thoughts without judgment, you create space between yourself and your worries.

Meditation also supports the production of feel-good brain chemicals like serotonin and dopamine. With regular practice, it can lift your mood, ease emotional distress, and help you feel more centered during treatment and recovery.[4]

▶ Mental Clarity

Meditation helps you notice emotions without being swept away by them. Various practices teach you to observe your feelings with gentleness and distance, so you can respond rather than react. This kind of emotional awareness builds resilience, allowing you to meet challenges with more steadiness and grace. Meditation also nurtures a mindset of acceptance, helping you face your illness with greater clarity and inner strength. These skills can make a meaningful difference as you navigate the emotional ups and downs of treatment.[5]

▶ Quality of Life

By easing stress, boosting immune function, relieving pain, and reducing anxiety and depression, meditation offers moments of peace in the midst of a difficult time. Regular practice can lift your mood, improve sleep, and offer a deeper sense of meaning. For many people, meditation becomes more than a coping tool—it becomes a way to reconnect with hope, healing, and inner strength.[6]

Meditation Practices for Healing and Recovery

▶ Mindfulness Meditation

Mindfulness meditation is one of the most widely practiced forms of meditation today. It involves tuning into the present moment—whether you're focusing on your breath, physical sensations, or emotions—without judgment. The goal isn't to clear your mind, but to gently observe your thoughts as they come and go. This kind of awareness builds emotional resilience and reduces stress, anxiety, and depression. By learning to meet each moment with curiosity and calm, mindfulness meditation helps you navigate life's challenges with greater ease.

Dr. Jon Kabat-Zinn, a molecular biologist at the University of Massachusetts Medical School, developed the Mindfulness-Based Stress Reduction (MBSR) program in 1979 to bring mindfulness into mainstream medicine. Since then, MBSR has become a widely used tool for helping people manage the physical and emotional side effects of cancer treatment. Today, MBSR and similar mindfulness programs are available around the world, both in person and online.

▶ Loving-Kindness Meditation (Metta)

Loving-kindness meditation—often called *Metta*—is about cultivating compassion and goodwill, starting with yourself and expanding outward. During this practice, you silently repeat simple phrases such as "May I be safe, may I be healthy, may I live with ease," and then extend those same wishes to others: loved ones, acquaintances, and even people you find challenging.

This meditation helps soften judgment and open your heart. Over time, it builds empathy and reduces feelings of anger, resentment, or isolation. For cancer patients, loving-kindness meditation can be especially comforting, helping them feel more connected to others and more supported from within.

▶ Body Scan Meditation

Body scan meditation gently guides your awareness through each part of your body, from your toes to the top of your head. The goal isn't to change anything, but simply to notice what's there—tingling, tension, warmth, or stillness—with curiosity and kindness.

This practice can be especially helpful if you're dealing with pain, fatigue, or trouble sleeping. By tuning into your body without judgment, you begin to recognize where you're holding stress and allow those areas to soften. Over time, the body scan helps deepen the mind-body connection, creating space for relaxation, healing, and a greater sense of presence.

How to Build a Daily Meditation Practice

A cancer diagnosis can feel like standing in the eye of a storm, with emotions and uncertainty swirling around you. In moments like these, finding stillness may seem nearly impossible. But meditation offers a way to pause, catch your breath, and return to yourself—even if only for a few minutes.

The beauty of meditation is its simplicity. You don't need a special cushion, incense, or an hour of free time. Just a quiet space, a few undisturbed minutes, and a willingness to show up as you are.

▶ Getting Started

- **Start small.** Try meditating for five to ten minutes a day. A short, consistent practice is more sustainable—and more powerful—than trying to do too much all at once.

- **Pick a peaceful spot.** Find a quiet, comfortable space where you won't be interrupted. This could be a corner of your bedroom, a cozy chair, or even a patch of sunlit grass.

- **Choose a time that works for you.** Some people prefer to meditate in the morning to set a calm tone for the day, while others use it to wind down before bed. Try both and see what feels best.

▶ Frequency and Duration

- **Aim for consistency.** A daily practice—even if it's just five minutes—can be more impactful than occasional longer sessions.

- **Work your way up.** As it gets easier, gradually increase your meditation time—from five minutes to ten, fifteen, twenty, or even longer if you like.

- **Let it fit your life.** Some days might be shorter, others longer. What matters most is showing up regularly, not perfectly.

▶ Practical Tips

- **Be kind to yourself.** Meditation is a practice. If your mind wanders, gently bring your attention back without judgment.

- **Use your breath.** Whether you're meditating or not, simply pausing to notice your breath can bring calm and clarity.

- **Pair it with what soothes you.** Try meditating after gentle yoga or a walk in nature or while listening to calming music. Combining the two can deepen your experience.

▶ Monitor Your Progress

- **Notice what shifts.** Pay attention to how you feel before and after meditating. You might start to see small changes in your mood, your sleep, or how you respond to stress.

- **Make it your own.** If a certain technique doesn't feel right, try another. There's no single right way to meditate—just the one that works best for you.

- **Stick with it.** Like any healing practice, meditation takes time. Some days it will come easily; other days, not so much. And that's OK. What matters most is showing up.

As more studies continue to highlight the benefits of meditation for cancer patients, medical facilities across the globe are integrating meditation into their cancer care programs.[7] Whether practiced alone or in a group, meditation offers a gentle yet powerful way to build resilience, calm the nervous system, and find peace in the midst of uncertainty. If you're new to meditation, consider exploring classes offered through your hospital or local community.

There are also many meditation apps available on iOS and Android devices, making it easy to practice meditation anytime, anywhere.

Meditation Apps for Cancer Support

You don't need to meditate alone—or figure it all out yourself. These apps offer guided meditations that can help you find calm, manage stress, and ease pain or anxiety during treatment. Many are easy to navigate and offer a range of free or low-cost options to help you get started.

- **Calm**
  Calm is one of the most widely used meditation apps, offering guided meditations for stress, anxiety, sleep, and pain. You'll also find breathing exercises, music, and soothing bedtime stories. Some content is free, though a subscription unlocks the full library.

- **Headspace**
  Headspace combines science-backed meditation practices with a friendly, approachable style. It offers programs for beginners and specific tracks for managing stress, anxiety, sleep, and even treatment-related fatigue. Like Calm, it requires a subscription for full access but offers some free options to start.

- **Insight Timer**
  Insight Timer features one of the largest collections of guided meditations, with thousands available for free. You'll find sessions on stress, sleep, pain, and emotional healing, along with mindfulness, loving-kindness, body scans, and guided imagery. The app also offers content created specifically for cancer patients and survivors—just type "cancer" into the search bar. A premium subscription unlocks extras like offline access and personalized tools.

- **Memorial Sloan Kettering Cancer Center's Meditation Resources**
  MSK offers a robust collection of free guided meditations specifically created for people living with cancer. You'll find sessions tailored to the newly diagnosed, those in treatment, and anyone managing stress, pain, or sleep challenges. You can stream or download them for offline use by visiting the Memorial Sloan Kettering Cancer Center website: www.mskcc.org/meditations.

Whether you're just beginning or returning to the practice, meditation can be a powerful companion throughout your cancer journey. Even a few minutes a day can help you breathe a little easier, feel a little calmer, and remember that peace is still possible—even now. Begin gently, with what feels right today. Follow what brings you peace or quiet curiosity. And allow yourself the kindness to grow your practice, one breath at a time.

Chapter 20

Guided Imagery

"The soul never thinks without a picture."
—ARISTOTLE, *De Anima (On the Soul)*

For centuries, people have turned to the imagination not just for escape, but for healing. Guided imagery draws on this time-honored healing tradition to calm the mind and strengthen the body. It's a meditative practice that uses visualization to create calming inner landscapes, supporting relaxation, emotional balance, and overall well-being.

Its roots run deep, stretching back to ancient civilizations. In Greece, philosophers like Hippocrates believed that imagination could influence both mind and body and that vivid mental imagery could influence physical responses and promote healing.

Dr. Martin Rossman, cofounder of the Academy for Guided Imagery and author of *Guided Imagery for Self-Healing*, has shown how various spiritual and cultural traditions—from Native American healers to Tibetan monks, Hindu sages, and practitioners of traditional Chinese medicine—have long relied on image-based practices to support physical and spiritual health.[1]

In the nineteenth century, hypnosis brought new attention to the power of imagery. It helped pave the way for Freud's psychoanalysis and Carl Jung's concept of "active imagination"—a technique that invites you to explore your unconscious mind by interacting with inner symbols, images, and emotions.

Today, guided imagery is used in all kinds of healthcare and therapeutic settings. In a typical session, you're gently led to picture vivid, calming scenes that tap into all your senses—sight, sound, smell, touch, and even taste—creating a rich, immersive experience. This kind of visualization can settle your nervous system, ease stress, and support your body's natural ability to heal.

It's also easier than ever to try. You can access guided imagery through mobile apps, audio tracks, YouTube videos, online classes, or even virtual and in-person support groups.

More and more, it's showing up in hospitals and clinics, too. Studies show that guided imagery can cut surgical complications in half, speed up hospital recovery times, relieve or prevent nausea caused by chemotherapy and radiation, reduce pain, and lessen anxiety and depression during treatment.[2]

After my diagnosis, I had the good fortune of meeting Dr. Rossman, whose practice was near my home in Marin County. Guided imagery helped me through some of the most challenging parts of my cancer treatment, including radiation, chemotherapy, and post-surgery recovery. I also relied on it during MRIs, which I found loud and claustrophobic. Visualizing the Volcano Rainforest Retreat on the Big Island of Hawaii helped make the unbearable bearable (the significance of this destination will be revealed in Chapter 25: Reiki).

How Guided Imagery Works

Guided imagery taps into the mind-body connection—the idea that what you imagine can influence how you feel, both physically and emotionally. Most practices rely on three key elements:

- **Visualization.** You create a mental picture of something calming or restorative, like a quiet forest, ocean waves, or your body repairing itself from within.
- **Relaxation.** As your focus deepens, your breathing slows, your muscles soften, and stress hormones like cortisol begin to drop.
- **Sensory engagement.** You draw on all five senses—imagining sights, sounds, scents, textures, and even tastes—to make the experience more vivid and real.

How Guided Imagery Can Help You

▶ Reduce Anxiety and Stress

Guided imagery provides a mental refuge—a safe, calming space where you can step away from fear and worry. Research shows that guided imagery is particularly beneficial for cancer patients undergoing chemotherapy, radiation, or surgery.[3] A study at Beth Israel Medical Center found that breast cancer patients who practiced guided imagery before and after radiation therapy experienced lower stress and anxiety levels.[4] Visualizing peaceful or healing imagery can help lower stress hormones like cortisol, creating a sense of calm that's been linked to better treatment outcomes.[5]

▶ Improve Pain Management

Guided imagery can shift how your brain processes pain. When paired with progressive muscle relaxation, it has been shown to significantly reduce pain, distress, anxiety, and depression compared to standard care.[6] By focusing on calming, healing images, you can reframe your perception of pain and activate your body's natural healing response.

▶ Enhance Immune Function

Patients with cancer often have weakened immune systems due to the disease and its treatments, making immune support essential. Research suggests that reducing stress through guided imagery and progressive muscle relaxation can enhance immune function by increasing natural killer cell activity—white blood cells that help fight illness—and by supporting other key indicators of immune health.[7]

▶ Alleviate Nausea and Vomiting

Chemotherapy-induced nausea and vomiting are among the most distressing side effects of cancer treatment. Research shows that guided imagery can be an effective, drug-free way to ease these symptoms. According to a study in the *Clinical Journal of Oncology Nursing*, guided imagery significantly reduced the severity of chemotherapy-induced nausea in cancer patients.[8] Patients who listened to guided imagery audio for twenty minutes daily reported notable reductions in both nausea and anxiety. Another study in the *Journal of Clinical Nursing* found that combining music therapy with visual imagery helped further relieve nausea, vomiting, and emotional distress.[9]

▶ Support Your Health Before and After Surgery

Research shows that guided imagery can be a valuable tool for patients undergoing surgery. Those who practiced it beforehand reported better quality of life both before and after their procedures. Guided imagery has also been shown to ease presurgical anxiety, reduce pain, and even shorten hospital stays, making it a powerful aid for both preparation and recovery.[10]

▶ Strengthen Your Emotional Well-Being

Cancer treatment can take a heavy emotional toll, often leading to feelings of depression, helplessness, and isolation. Guided imagery helps counter these effects by fostering a sense of empowerment and optimism. Visualizing positive outcomes—like a tumor shrinking—can cultivate hope and resilience. Research shows that people who practice guided imagery often report improved mood, greater emotional balance, and a renewed sense of hope.[11]

▶ Enhance Quality of Life

The ultimate goal of guided imagery is to help you feel better—physically, emotionally, and spiritually. When woven into a larger treatment plan, it can give you a greater sense of control and hope, making the overall experience more manageable and, often, more positive.

Where to Find Guided Imagery Practitioners

If you're interested in exploring guided imagery with a trained practitioner, there are a variety of options available to suit your needs.

- **Hospitals and cancer centers.** Many major cancer centers—like Memorial Sloan Kettering and MD Anderson—offer guided imagery through their integrative oncology programs. If you're receiving care at a medical center, check with their integrative medicine department to see if they have certified practitioners on staff.

- **Certified guided imagery networks.** The Academy for Guided Imagery offers resources and training for guided imagery practitioners. You can find certified professionals by visiting www.acadgi.com/directory.

Guided imagery is more than just a relaxation technique. It's a way to shift how you experience illness and healing. By tapping into your mind's ability to influence your body, it helps you take a more active, empowered role in your care. Whether you're using it to ease anxiety, reduce fatigue, manage pain, improve sleep, relieve nausea, lift your mood, or support your emotional well-being, guided imagery is a gentle, drug-free complement to traditional cancer treatment.

Chapter 21

Somatic Yoga

"Somatic yoga is a process of reeducating
the body and mind to move with ease
and efficiency, enhancing awareness
and promoting well-being."
—ELEANOR CRISWELL, *How Yoga Works:
Introduction to Somatic Yoga*

Somatic yoga is a gentle yet powerful practice that helped restore my mind, body, and spirit during recovery. I was introduced to it by JeanMarie Murphy, founder of Taking Refuge, a local clinic that supported people undergoing cancer treatment. A seasoned healer and teacher, JeanMarie has guided mindfulness and body-awareness practices for more than thirty years.

As a somatic yoga student, I came to understand that chronic tension reflects the way we carry our lived experiences—in our muscles, our thoughts, and our emotions. Drawing from her deep knowledge of somatics, anatomy, physiology, and neurobiology, JeanMarie helps students gently unwind the layers of trauma held in their bodies.

To share what I learned, I asked JeanMarie a few questions. This chapter presents her answers—in her own words.

What Is Somatic Yoga?

JEANMARIE: Somatic yoga is a mindful relaxation practice that releases muscular tension, enhances circulation, increases body awareness, and improves neural communication between your brain and all your muscles, organs, and glands. Daily practice supports your autonomic nervous system, resulting in a more positive mindset, improved cardio and circulatory health, reduced inflammation, and enhanced sleep.

Consciously or unconsciously, your body keeps track of and stores every physical, emotional, and mental experience. In combination, these experiences leave a trace or an imprint within your body that ultimately affects the way you move in the world. Somatic yoga helps your body to unwind and release chronically held tensions and any emotional habits that no longer serve you, allowing you to live more fully in the present moment.

Somatic yoga nourishes your entire nervous system, improving communication between your brain and brain stem (your central nervous system) and the neural networks that deliver information to your muscles, organs, and glands (your peripheral nervous system). It supports the innate intelligence of the body with an intention of activating the side of your nervous system that is focused on relaxation. Instead of forcing your body to assume a yoga posture, somatic yoga gently coaxes your body into fluid movement that nurtures and supports it.

What Role Does Breath Play in Somatic Yoga?

JEANMARIE: In somatic yoga, we consciously synchronize all movement with our breath. When we move into a posture, we exhale. When we return to our starting position, we inhale. With each inhalation, we nourish our body with fresh oxygen. With each exhalation, we experience a deep release of chronic tension, while also releasing carbon dioxide.

How Can Somatic Yoga Support Cancer Treatment?

JEANMARIE: Yoga, as a therapeutic somatic practice, holds great potential for healing. It can teach you about the innate intelligence of the body and its natural capacity to heal. When you actively cultivate a daily practice of relaxation, you simultaneously reduce your level of stress and the damaging effects of elevated stress hormones circulating in your bloodstream.

Somatic yoga can also help you prepare for surgery and recover more quickly afterword. As you release chronically held tension and learn how to relax, you're enhancing circulation throughout your body. By gently reintroducing movement after surgery, you can increase your circulation and flexibility in the affected areas.

What Are Your Favorite Somatic Yoga Movements?

JEANMARIE: When practiced together, the Knee-Down Twist, Pelvic Rocking, and the Pelvic Clock will support your structural muscles to release deeply held mental and emotional tensions that lead to chronic holding patterns. Ultimately, these exercises can improve neural communication between your brain and all your muscles, organs, and glands while teaching your body how to relax.

KNEE-DOWN TWIST

Think of this movement as a lullaby for your spine.

1. Lie on your back with your eyes closed, and stretch your arms out on the floor at shoulder level with your palms facing down.
2. Bend your knees and place your feet on the floor so that your knees and feet are about hip-width apart, a comfortable distance from your buttocks. This posture is called semi-supine.

3. Take a deep breath in, and as you exhale, guide your knees to the left. Inhale them back to center, and then exhale guiding your knees to the right. Continue exhaling to the side and inhaling to center, synchronizing your body movement with the movement of your breath.
4. When comfortable with your synchronization, begin to add the movement of your neck and head. As you exhale your knees to the left, roll your neck and head to the right. Inhale everything back to center. Then as you exhale, guide your knees to the right, and roll your neck and head to the left. Continue for at least two minutes.
5. When you feel complete, rest for a few moments in semi-supine. Observe how your body feels different from when you started. Then move on to Pelvic Rocking.

PELVIC ROCKING

Think of this movement as an opportunity to enhance the relationship between your upper and lower body.

1. Close your eyes and allow your teeth to part so your jaw can relax.
2. Begin to arch your lower back off the floor using your lower back muscles. Feel your abdominal muscles lengthen as your lower back muscles contract.
3. Now reverse your movement by gently curling your lower back using your abdominal muscles. As your abdominal muscles contract, feel your lower back muscles lengthening and making firm contact with the floor. Your tailbone should be slightly pointing up toward the ceiling.
4. Continue alternating between arching and curling while keeping your buttocks on the floor. In this exercise, your lower back muscles and abdominal muscles are learning to work together as a team.

5. When you are comfortable with the movement, you can begin to synchronize your movement to your breath; inhale as you arch and exhale as you curl. Enjoy for at least two minutes. When you feel complete, rest for a few moments, observe your body, and then move to the Pelvic Clock.

THE PELVIC CLOCK

Think of this movement as an opportunity to create greater communication between your abdominal muscles and lower back muscles.

1. Place an imaginary clock underneath your sacrum. When you arch your lower back, your tailbone is pointed toward six o'clock, and when you curl your lower back, the top of your sacrum is pointing at noon. So, with your previous movement—pelvic rocking—you are moving between six o'clock and noon.
2. For the pelvic clock, start at noon and slowly roll over to the back of your left hip, which would be three o'clock, rolling down to six o'clock (as when you arch), and then roll up and over to the back of your right hip, which would be nine o'clock, and then back up to the top of your sacrum and noon (as when you curl). Move clockwise—from noon to three o'clock, to six o'clock, to nine o'clock—in a slow, peaceful, circular manner for five complete cycles. Now reverse the clock: Move from noon to nine o'clock, to six o'clock, then three o'clock for five complete cycles.
3. When you are complete, be still for a few breaths while observing your lower back and belly. Feel your body relaxing into the present moment. Complete your practice with five to ten minutes of lying on the floor or sitting in meditation. Then enjoy a full glass of water.

Through my journey with cancer, somatic yoga became an invaluable part of my healing process, offering a gentle yet powerful way to reconnect with my body, mind, and spirit. JeanMarie's teachings helped me release deeply held tension—both physical and emotional—and regain a sense of control over my body. As I navigated the challenges of treatment, somatic yoga reminded me of the body's innate intelligence and capacity for healing, guiding me toward a path of relaxation, recovery, and renewed hope.

I hope these practices inspire you to explore the possibilities of somatic yoga as you begin—or continue—your own journey to wellness.

Chapter 22

Jin Shin Jyutsu

"The part can never be well unless the whole is well."
—PLATO, *Charmides*

Shortly after I was diagnosed with breast cancer, I began working with a Jin Shin Jyutsu practitioner through my cancer center's Integrative Healing Program. Jin Shin Jyutsu was a gift I might never have discovered were it not for my cancer diagnosis. What began as an introduction to a complementary therapy quickly became a meaningful part of my care.

By day, while undergoing chemo, it kept nausea at bay. By night, it helped me overcome anxiety and insomnia. During radiation, it helped me ward off burns and fatigue. And after my surgeries in San Francisco and New Orleans, a practitioner visited my hospital room to reduce pain and speed my recovery—a gesture that eased both body and spirit.

Jin Shin Jyutsu (pronounced Jin-SHIN-Jit-Soo) is a Japanese healing art developed in the early 20th century by Jiro Murai, a philosopher who is said to have recovered from a life-threatening illness. His experience led to a lifelong study of ancient healing philosophies, which he synthesized into what is now known as Jin Shin Jyutsu.

Though modern in form, the practice draws on ancient Eastern concepts, including those found in the *Huangdi Neijing* (*The Yellow Emperor's Classic of Internal Medicine*), a foundational Chinese medical text compiled between 475 BCE and 220 CE. Both emphasize the flow of vital energy through the body and the importance of maintaining balance across physical, emotional, and spiritual dimensions of health. The practice was introduced to the United States around 1965 by Murai's student Mary Burmeister.

This gentle, noninvasive healing art uses the light placement of fingers on specific points of the body to balance energy and restore well-being. As a complement to conventional care, Jin Shin Jyutsu helps ease chronic symptoms. When practiced regularly, it can calm the nervous system, relieve pain, combat fatigue and insomnia, enhance emotional stability, and support immune function. It has also been known to shorten healing time after surgery. In short, Jin Shin Jyutsu promotes optimal health and well-being by harnessing the body's natural ability to heal.

Jin Shin Jyutsu is a valuable complement to conventional medicine. It works with twenty-six "safety energy locks" located along pathways that guide the flow of energy through the body. When one or more of these pathways becomes blocked, energy can stagnate, initially affecting a localized area and, over time, the entire system. By gently holding specific combinations of these energy locks, you can help restore balance to your mind, body, and spirit.

Sessions typically last about an hour and involve no massage, muscle manipulation, or substances. Practitioners gently place their fingertips—over clothing—on specific safety energy locks to awaken and harmonize energy flow. Jin Shin Jyutsu can be safely used alongside both conventional medicine and complementary therapies.

How to Practice Jin Shin Jyutsu on Yourself and Others

When practicing Jin Shin Jyutsu, remember: You can't do it wrong. If your hands move intuitively rather than following the exact instructions, trust that your body knows what it needs. Jin Shin Jyutsu activates the body's innate healing intelligence, gently guiding energy to where it's needed most. Practicing a little each day is often more effective than doing a lot once in a while. If you engage with it daily—even for just a few minutes—you're likely to experience a meaningful difference.

▶ Main Central Vertical Flow

This foundational sequence activates the body's primary energy system through a series of hand positions. It can amplify the benefits of your healing regimen and help minimize side effects from medications and treatments like chemotherapy and radiation. Practicing it first thing in the morning is especially effective for setting a grounded, balanced tone for the day ahead.

You can perform this sequence lying down or seated.

STEP 1: Place your right hand on the top of your head.

STEP 2: With your left hand, move down the center of your body, touching each of the following points for two to three minutes:

- Center of forehead
- Tip of nose
- Hollow of the throat (just above the collarbone)
- Center of chest
- Solar plexus (base of the ribcage)
- Two inches above the navel
- Two inches below the navel
- Front of pubic bone

STEP 3: Move your right hand from the top of your head to your tailbone.

▶ Anxiety and Depression

Wrap your opposite hand gently around each finger for two minutes per finger, on both hands (twenty minutes total).

▶ Backache

Place your fingertips in the crease where your torso meets your upper thighs. Place your right fingertips in the right crease and your left fingertips in the left crease. This can be done sitting, standing, or lying down. Hold for fifteen minutes.

▶ Compromised Immune System

Place your left hand on your left shoulder with your fingertips slightly down the upper back next to the spine. Lightly place your right thumb on top of each fingernail (index through pinkie) for one to two minutes each. Reverse hands and repeat both steps. **Total time:** ten to twenty minutes.

This is also an invaluable preventative treatment for colds and flus, especially when you're around contagious people.

▶ Fatigue

Place your palms on the sides of your head with your fingertips touching at the crown. Hold for five to ten minutes. (Twenty minutes is optimal.)

▶ Headache

While seated, cross your wrists, and press your hands gently into the insides of your opposite knees. Hold for ten to twenty minutes.

▶ Heart Conditions and Poor Circulation

Wrap the fingers of one hand around the pinkie of the other. Switch hands and repeat. Total time: ten to fifteen minutes.

For heart support. Place your right hand at the base of your left ribs and your left hand on the thumb side of your right forearm at the elbow. This hold is most effective when done on this side only. However, if it would be more comfortable for you, place your left hand at the base of your right ribs and your right hand on the thumb side of your left forearm at the elbow. Total time: ten minutes.

For improved circulation. Place your left hand in the crease of your left groin and your right hand on the center of your left foot arch. Then switch sides, placing your right hand in the crease of your right groin and your left hand on the center of your right foot arch. Total time: ten minutes.

▶ Hot Flashes

Place three fingers of your right hand on the right side of your neck, just below the ear. With your left hand, place your left thumb pad over the nail of your left ring finger. Hold each position simultaneously for five to ten minutes.

▶ Insomnia

VARIATION 1: Gently wrap your fingers around your thumb, then pinkie, on both hands for five minutes each.

VARIATION 2: Touch your right palm to your solar plexus (just below your ribcage) and use your left hand to hold your right thumb, then pinkie, for two minutes each. Repeat the same sequence with your left palm touching your solar plexus. Total time: eight minutes.

▶ Lymphedema

To reduce swelling, use the hand opposite the affected arm. For example, if you have swelling in your right arm, cup your right underarm with your left hand, touching the outer edge of your right shoulder blade with your left fingertips. At the same time, with your right hand, touch the fingernails of the ring finger, then the pinkie finger, for one to two minutes each. Total time: two to four minutes.

▶ Mouth Sores

VARIATION 1: Place your palms on the backs of your calves. Hold for three to five minutes.

VARIATION 2: Place the palm side of your fingers or the back of your hand over your kidneys (at the base of the ribs, beside the spine). Hold for up to twenty minutes.

▶ Nausea

VARIATION 1: Cross your hands at the wrists and apply slight pressure two inches above the inside of your knees. Hold for ten to twenty minutes.

VARIATION 2: During chemotherapy, wrap the fingers of your right hand around your left index finger and hold for three minutes. Repeat with the other hand. Total time: ten to twenty minutes.

▶ PMS and Menopause

Place one hand on the back of your neck, applying light pressure. With your other hand, place your thumb over your ring fingernail. Total time: Hold for five to ten minutes, then switch hands and repeat.

▶ Radiation Burns

After each radiation session, to help prevent burning, place the palm of your right hand on top of your left hand, holding both hands together one inch above the radiated area. This draws out excess heat and can ease discomfort. This method works on other burns as well. Total time: five to ten minutes.

Tip: To reduce radiation side effects, practice the Main Central Vertical Flow immediately before and after radiation.

▶ Surgery Recovery

This is called Opposite Fingers and Toes. The description may sound complicated, but it's easy once you start. To speed healing and reduce recovery time after surgery, have a friend or family member help with this. Have your helper sit or stand at your left or right side. They begin with the hand closest to yours, holding your thumb and your opposite-side pinkie toe simultaneously for one minute. For example, if they're holding your right thumb, they would also hold your left pinkie toe with their other hand at the same time. Then continue to the next adjacent finger and toe pair, and so on, holding each set simultaneously for one minute. Next, have them reach across to your other hand and begin again with the thumb and pinkie toe, working through each adjacent pair for one minute, as before. Ten finger-toe sets at one minute each equals a total time of ten minutes. For best results, repeat daily for up to a week after surgery.

Jin Shin Jyutsu has been a guiding light in my healing journey, offering me an empowering way to actively participate in my own recovery. Its gentle yet transformative techniques have helped me manage the physical side effects of cancer treatment, support my emotional well-being, and harness my body's natural ability to heal. Whether you're navigating the challenges of cancer or simply seeking relief from the stresses of daily life, Jin Shin Jyutsu provides a calming path to greater vitality and well-being.

It continues to be an essential part of my self-care, and I hope these simple yet powerful practices become a meaningful part of yours, too.

To learn more or locate certified practitioners in the United States or internationally, visit www.jsjsmb.org. For clear and accessible guidance on self-practice, I recommend *The Touch of Healing* by Alice Burmeister and Tom Monte.

Chapter 23

Qigong

> "Qigong is the art and science of refining and cultivating internal energy."
> KEN COHEN, *The Way of Qigong*

Qigong (pronounced chee-GONG), which literally means "working with the energy of life," is an integrated mind-body healing practice that has been used with remarkable results in China for thousands of years. Today, this term encompasses more than 3,600 distinct styles practiced around the world.

According to Ken Cohen, renowned Qigong master and author of *The Way of Qigong: The Art and Science of Chinese Energy Healing*, "the Chinese have long treasured Qigong for its effectiveness both in healing and in preventing disease, and more recently they have used it in conjunction with modern medicine to cure cancer, immune system disorders, and other life-threatening conditions."[1]

In the United States, many cancer hospitals now incorporate Qigong into their integrative medicine programs to support patients during and after treatment. Notable institutions offering Qigong include Memorial Sloan Kettering Cancer Center in

New York and MD Anderson Cancer Center in Houston. If you're interested in exploring Qigong, check with your medical center's integrative medicine program to see if it is available.

While in search of a Qigong instructor, I was introduced to Shirley Dockstader, an accredited ChiLel Qigong teacher who has taught ancient Eastern healing arts for more than thirty years. During my cancer treatment, I found her classes to be a joyful refuge—a place I could return to each week to gently calm my frayed nerves while also uplifting my energy and spirit. Here, Shirley shares her unique understanding of Qigong in our interview.

The Origin of Qigong

SHIRLEY: According to Chinese legend, the rains poured down relentlessly on the ancient people of the Tao Tang Tribe, bringing season after season of floods. The people began to despair and sicken as the constant wet and cold invaded their joints, tissues, and dispositions. The tribal leaders called on healing shamans for help. They knew the stagnation in the fields had also penetrated the landscape of the people's bodies. The shamans showed the members of this ancient tribe how to deepen their breath and how to move and dance in partnership with their breath. These movements were expansive, rhythmic, and fluid. This shamanic dance (the *Da Wu*) moved the sluggish fluids in tribe members' bodies, which improved their health and ultimately lifted their spirits.

How Qigong Works

SHIRLEY: The healing art and science of Qigong uses six main methods to cultivate *qi* (or chi, pronounced chee): alignment, breath, movement, sound, visualization, and the attention of the mind. All of these practices help bring balance and harmony between what is within us and what surrounds us.

Qigong is based on the principles of Chinese medicine and its understanding of the flow of life-giving energy (chi) through a network of channels called meridians. Each of the twelve major meridians is associated with the function of the organ for which it is named.

All forms of Qigong share:

- **Alignment.** Channels must be open for anything to flow through them. Whether you are seated, standing, or even lying in bed, you want your body to be opened and relaxed.

- **Breath.** Nature gave our breath the power to move our internal waterways, just as the wind moves ocean currents. We are about 75 percent water, and water is the key circulator of information and energy (chi) for the cells. Breath is chi in its most accessible form.

- **Intention.** In this ancient practice, there is no separation between heart and mind. Seeking wholeness for our body, heart, mind, and spirit, we visualize an abundant flow of chi, a healthy body, and a calm state of mind—balancing the world inside us with the universe that surrounds us.

How Qigong Can Help You Heal

SHIRLEY: Research in China provides considerable evidence of the benefits of Qigong to cancer patients. According to traditional Chinese medicine and Qigong, cancer indicates the stagnation of vital life force energy (chi), blood, and other bodily fluids. Because Qigong practices are designed specifically to dispel stagnation and strengthen the flow of blood and chi, in China, Qigong takes place alongside Western medicine in the treatment of cancer.

When you bring yourself into a Qigong state of deep relaxation and tranquility, your body's natural healing system is activated. In this state—when your cells are fully oxygenated and your circulation of blood and lymph is improved—you will benefit by having more energy, better concentration and memory, improved appetite, less pain, and more satisfying sleep.

Four Energizing Movements for People of Any Age

SHIRLEY:

▶ Accessing Your Chi

- Sitting or standing, connect your feet to the earth, then imagine sending imaginary roots from your feet down into the ground. Relax your hips and slightly tuck in your tailbone.
- Drop your shoulders and pull your shoulder blades toward each other in the back. This will open your heart and thymus.
- Lift from the crown of your head. Slightly tuck in your chin, widening the base of your skull. Now place your tongue where your upper teeth and gums meet. This is called the Taoist Inner Smile. It has an immediate soothing effect on the thymus and the whole body.
- Drop your attention into this alignment. To melt all tension, imagine opening from the inside out through your skin into the space around you. Notice the spaciousness you feel inside.

▶ The Invisible Chi Ball

In this relaxed and open state, bring your palms together and rub them vigorously against each other until they are quite warm.

Then, slowly pull them apart at the level of your heart, as if holding an invisible ball of energy. Close your eyes and bring your attention to the space between your palms. Open and close your hands very slowly. You may notice some resistance between them, possibly some sensation in your hands. Or you may not. But if you are thinking chi ball, it is there. Where the mind goes, the chi follows.

▶ Belly Breathing

Our abdomen is the energy center in our body. It is also known as *dan tien* in meditative and exercise techniques such as Qigong, the martial art of t'ai chi, and in traditional Chinese medicine. Nature gave our breath the power to move nourishing waves of chi from this vital source of energy out into our cells and organs, calming and balancing the nervous system and helping our lymphatic system remove waste.

Holding the chi ball between your hands, breathe in slowly as you open your hands to the side, widening the chi ball between your palms, expanding the space in your abdomen. Relax completely as your breath goes out and your chi ball condenses back to your center. Making sure your shoulders are relaxed and down, repeat opening and closing the chi ball in a comfortable and relaxed rhythm. Visualize the waves of chi coming in and going out in the sea of chi in your abdomen, carrying nourishing energy to the far shores of your body. This simple breathing practice can also be done lying down.

▶ Wild Goose Spreads Its Wings—Thymus Expansion

In this expansive movement, the chest opens wide with the breath, stimulating the master gland of the immune system—the thymus gland. Besides improving immune function, this whole-body movement gets blood, lymph, and chi circulating efficiently.

Still holding the chi ball, step forward slightly on your left foot. As you take a deep breath in, shift your weight forward and open your arms wide to the side, feeling your heart and thymus open and expand with the breath. Pause in the fullness of the breath, then shift your weight to your back leg as you bring the chi ball back together in front of your body on a long and complete exhale. Immediately open your arms wide again, bringing fresh chi and abundant oxygen into the thymus gland. Repeat several times on each side.

End your Qigong practice by opening your arms wide to the side, embracing a big chi ball, and drawing it in to your center. Then, with eyes closed, take a moment to nourish the chi that you've cultivated in your center.

Qigong offers a path to healing and resilience that can complement traditional cancer treatments by enhancing physical vitality, calming the mind, and restoring inner balance. Whether you practice on your own or under the guidance of a skilled instructor, incorporating Qigong into your routine can support your body's natural healing processes and provide a sense of calm and empowerment amid the challenges of treatment. Embrace these simple yet powerful movements to cultivate energy, foster relaxation, and nourish your well-being.

Chapter 24

Feldenkrais

"No part of the body can be moved without all the others being affected."
—MOSHE FELDENKRAIS,
Body and Mature Behavior

The Feldenkrais Method was developed by Dr. Moshe Feldenkrais, a Russian-born physicist, mechanical and electrical engineer, judo expert, and educator. His approach draws on principles of physics and biomechanics, combined with a deep understanding of how we learn through movement.

This gentle, innovative approach helps you explore how you move and understand the connections between your nervous system, muscles, skeleton, and your responses to the world around you. As you practice, you may notice greater flexibility, easier movement, better coordination, and an overall sense of well-being.

Feldenkrais (pronounced FELL-den-krice) can be especially helpful during cancer recovery. The movements are gentle and can be done while you're sitting, standing, or lying down—so you can still participate even when your body feels fragile or limited.

I was first introduced to Feldenkrais after my body had been traumatized by a bilateral mastectomy and, eight months later, reconstructive surgery. I felt as though I had been divided into two disconnected halves, each carrying its own pain and limitations. The upper half was compromised by my mastectomy and the removal of eighteen lymph nodes under my right arm. Scar tissue from the mastectomy limited movement in my neck, ribs, arms, and upper torso. The lower half of my body was compromised by the reconstructive surgery, which left me with an incision stretching from hip to hip across my abdomen. My goal was to rid my body of the feeling that it was no longer whole.

After my first appointment at a local clinic, I felt a glimmer of hope. By the end of the session, I distinctly remember feeling taller, with a newfound sense of spaciousness and mobility in my ribs, shoulders, neck, and arms.

With this kind of progress, I committed to weekly treatments for several months. Through repeated sessions, my once estranged body began to feel understood and move more comfortably. Finally, the invisible and almost indescribable issues from my surgeries were getting the attention they so desperately needed.

How Feldenkrais Rewires the Brain

In 1949, Moshe Feldenkrais proposed that the brain could reorganize itself by forming new connections—a concept now known as neuroplasticity. He taught people to stimulate their senses through very small movements that helped their brains form new neural pathways—what he referred to as "brain maps."

He called his classes Awareness Through Movement (ATM) lessons, and through these lessons, he helped adults recovering from strokes as well as children with cerebral palsy or autism. Feldenkrais's goal: "What I'm after isn't flexible bodies, but flexible brains. What I'm after is to restore each person to their human dignity."[1]

His words rang true for me. I felt that sense of dignity returning as I reconnected with my body.

How the Feldenkrais Method Can Help You

One of the things I love about the Feldenkrais Method is that almost anyone can do it, even if they're unable to exercise in a traditional way. It's particularly beneficial for those recovering from injury or illness, as it helps restore function without causing strain. Awareness Through Movement lessons teach you to reduce your effort whenever possible, and to understand that errors are essential and there is no "right" way to move—only better ways.

Many people who practice Feldenkrais report meaningful improvements in how they feel and move. Some of the most common benefits include:

- Reduced musculoskeletal pain
- Greater ease of motion
- Deeper relaxation and fuller breathing
- Enhanced vitality
- Improved emotional well-being and comfort

How to Practice the Feldenkrais Method at Home

These movements help increase awareness and mobility, encouraging gentle, nonstrenuous exercise during recovery.

- **Spinal twist.** Lie on your back with knees bent, feet flat. Gently lower both knees to one side, then the other, slowly exploring your range of motion.
- **Hip circles.** Stand and gently circle your hips, as though tracing a wide, gentle circle with your pelvis.
- **Rolling like a ball.** Sit with your knees hugged to your chest. Gently rock back and forth, feeling how your body responds to the movement.
- **Lifting and lowering the head.** Lie on your back and gently lift your head off the floor, then lower it back down slowly, focusing on smoothness and ease of movement.
- **Jaw relaxation.** Sit comfortably, place your tongue on the roof of your mouth, and gently open and close your jaw, feeling the tension release.

How to Practice the Feldenkrais Method with a Practitioner

Feldenkrais work is done either in groups or one-on-one. Group sessions involve verbal instruction from a Feldenkrais teacher, who leads participants through a series of movements while sitting, lying on the floor, or standing. A lesson typically lasts between thirty and sixty minutes.

There are approximately six thousand certified practitioners of this method worldwide. To find a qualified practitioner, visit the Feldenkrais Guild of North America: www.feldenkrais.com.

The Feldenkrais Method takes a gentle, respectful approach to movement. It meets your body where it is and guides it toward greater ease and freedom. Whether you explore it on your own or work with a skilled practitioner, Feldenkrais can help you restore a sense of wholeness and vitality during recovery.

Chapter 25

Reiki

> "There is more wisdom in your body
> than in your deepest philosophy."
> —FRIEDRICH NIETZSCHE, *Thus Spoke Zarathustra*

The silver lining of my surgeon's impulsive lumpectomy was a rare two-week pause before chemo—an unexpected breath between shock and treatment. During that time, my husband had a conference scheduled on the Big Island of Hawaii, and since I didn't have to begin treatment right away, he invited me to join him. It was a bittersweet trip, shadowed by everything that lay ahead. But after the conference ended, my husband surprised me with the perfect remedy for the quiet dread I couldn't shake: the Volcano Rainforest Retreat.

After driving for hours, we were welcomed with open arms by the gracious owners, Kathleen and Peter, who led us through the lush rainforest to our private, Japanese-inspired sanctuary. Our hexagonal cedar studio, with its floor-to-ceiling windows, shifted my mood the moment we arrived. Just steps from our front door, we discovered a traditional Japanese soaking tub nestled between giant ferns and bamboo. This magical place would soon become my soul's refuge—a quiet haven I'd find myself returning to in my mind during claustrophobic MRIs and endless rounds of chemo and radiation.

To our surprise, we discovered that Kathleen and Peter were not only former Bay Area residents, but also renowned psychotherapists. As fate would have it, Kathleen was an experienced Reiki healer as well. On our final day, she generously offered me a session to help calm my body and spirit as I prepared to begin chemotherapy.

As I lay fully clothed on a futon, Kathleen gently held her hands a few inches above me, explaining that Reiki (pronounced RAY-kee) is a Japanese word meaning "universal life energy." She explained that Reiki doesn't heal directly but gently channels energy to support your body's natural healing response. During that hour, I felt a sacred connection—to Kathleen, to her energy work, and to the Volcano Rainforest Retreat itself. When the session ended, I walked away with a calm, quiet confidence that I would be all right.

That first session gave me a glimpse into Reiki's healing potential. Over time, I learned more about its origins and its growing recognition within modern healthcare. Developed in the early twentieth century by Japanese Buddhist and spiritual teacher Mikao Usui, Reiki was introduced to the United States in the 1930s and has steadily gained popularity ever since. This energy-based healing practice is rooted in the belief that practitioners can channel life-force energy through their hands to support the body's natural ability to heal.

Although I didn't engage with Reiki regularly during treatment—I was immersed in somatic yoga, Jin Shin Jyutsu, Qigong, and Feldenkrais—that first session stayed with me. It introduced me to a healing approach I would come to appreciate more deeply in the years that followed.

While more research is needed to fully understand how Reiki

produces its healing effects, both early studies and personal experiences like mine suggest that Reiki can offer meaningful relief from the challenges of cancer treatment—fatigue, anxiety, depression, nausea, and pain—while also improving overall quality of life.[1]

Whether you're undergoing chemotherapy, radiation, or surgery, Reiki can become a trusted companion on your path to healing. You don't need training or experience to begin—just a willingness to place your hands, breathe, and be present. You may feel warmth or tingling—or nothing at all. Either way, trust that your body is receiving what it needs.

The following self-guided sequence can be used anytime you need comfort, calm, or clarity.

To practice Reiki on yourself, place your hands directly on, or just above, any area that feels tender, tense, or in need of attention. To start, move your hands to your chest, over your heart, and breathe deeply, allowing your body to relax fully. Visualize healing energy flowing into your body, filling every cell with warmth and calm. Notice any warmth, tingling, or sensations beneath your hands. Hold for at least three to five minutes—or longer, if it feels good.

Next, place your hands on your lower belly, just below your navel, and hold for three to five minutes. This area, known as the *hara* in Japanese healing traditions, is considered the body's energetic center of balance and vitality. It is believed to be the seat of inner strength, intuition, and grounding. By holding your hands over the hara during Reiki practice, you tap into a deep well of healing energy, promoting stability, relaxation, and overall well-being.

Now, gently place your hands over your eyes or forehead as you take deep, calming breaths. Again, hold for three to five minutes, allowing your mind to quiet and your body to absorb the healing energy.

To close your session, bring your hands back to your heart and take a few slow, steady breaths to return to the present moment. You might want to silently thank your body for everything it's doing to support you right now. Then, set an intention—to carry this sense of calm and balance with you as you move through your day.

Reiki may seem subtle, but its impact is gaining wider recognition. As science continues to explore the mind-body connection, practices like Reiki are becoming more common in mainstream cancer care—even at leading institutions like MD Anderson, Memorial Sloan Kettering, and Mayo Clinic. It's also recognized by the National Center for Complementary and Integrative Health (NCCIH) as an energy-based therapy, which speaks to its growing acceptance in both medical and research communities.

Though I didn't return to Reiki much during treatment—I was drawn to other practices that felt more accessible at the time—my first experience with it stayed with me. It wasn't dramatic or life-changing, but it gave me something I hadn't known I needed: a quiet sense of trust in my body again. Even though it was carrying cancer, I could still feel my body's strength—its ability to support and heal me as I faced the challenges ahead.

In the months that followed—through chemo, radiation, and all the unknowns—I often found myself thinking back to that moment: lying still in that rainforest studio, Kathleen's hands hovering above me, and a quiet calm that rose from deep within. It reminded me that healing isn't always about fixing what's wrong. It can begin with simply feeling safe in your own body again.

Whether received from a skilled practitioner or practiced in the quiet of your own home, Reiki can be a gentle invitation to trust your body's ability to heal—one breath at a time.

If you'd like to explore Reiki with a certified practitioner in your area, visit:

- International Association of Reiki Professionals (IARP): www.iarp.org
- International Center for Reiki Training (ICRT): www.reiki.org

Chapter 26

Healing Affirmations

"All that we are is the result of
what we have thought."
—BUDDHA, *Dhammapada*

Affirmations are a meditative tool that can help you tap into—and strengthen—your inner resilience. During treatment, I began each morning by choosing one before I even got out of bed. I'd take a deep breath, say it slowly out loud, and let the words settle within me.

I found them especially helpful during chemo and radiation; before surgery; during MRIs; while traveling to medical appointments; upon waking; and before bedtime. Feel free to create your own—personalized affirmations are often the most powerful.

You may want to write a few on 3x5 cards to keep by your bedside or desk. I often carried one in my purse so it was easy to reach for throughout the day. You can also store them on your phone for a quick reminder whenever you need a moment of calm or encouragement.

Below are many of the affirmations that supported me throughout my journey. Most I created myself; others are mantras I adapted to nurture my healing.

Gratitude & Grounding

I am loved and I am safe.

Love is at the heart of my healing.

Love surrounds me, protects me, and fills me with peace.

I embrace myself with love and compassion.

I am anchored in the present moment,
finding peace in the here and now.

Everything is going to work out even better than I can imagine.

I feel deeply grounded and embraced
by a profound sense of well-being.

I am filled with gratitude for all that is good in my life.

Physical & Emotional Healing

I forgive my body and embrace its healing.

I embrace and accept my body exactly as it is.

My healing has already begun.

With each breath I take, I am healing every level of my being.

I inhale love. I exhale fear.

I trust my body's innate ability to heal and restore balance.

I listen with love to my body's messages.

My body is continually working to support my healing.

With each passing day, I move closer to healing and wholeness.

Growth and transformation continue to
unfold in unexpected ways.

Every day, I grow stronger in body, mind, and spirit.

Visualizations

I am surrounded by angels who will
guide me through this process.

I stand on a majestic mountain, facing my
challenges with clarity, strength, and courage.

Beneath a cascading waterfall,
I release tension, illness, and worry.

Golden sunlight streams through every cell in my body,
renewing my energy and vitality.

An army of tiny brooms sweeps through my body,
clearing away every last cancer cell.

My cancer is floating away in a big black balloon.

Today, I will rise from my basement to my virtual penthouse, where the air is fresh and my mind is clear.

As I close my eyes, I am cradled into deep, restorative sleep.

Self-Empowerment in Medical Settings

I feel safe and supported in the hands of skilled and compassionate caregivers.

I am my own best advocate, confidently navigating my care with clarity and strength.

I ask the right questions and make informed decisions about my treatment.

I understand that chemo brain is real, and I extend compassion to my mind as it heals.

I deeply appreciate the care, dedication, and expertise of my medical team.

Strength & Resilience

My cancer does not define me.

I am strong, centered, and calm.

I approach my healing one day at a time.

I choose to free myself from destructive fears and doubts.

I have the strength and courage to navigate
any challenge that comes my way.

I am willing to believe that something else is possible.

I will go through this with an open mind.

I welcome new and creative ways to support my healing.

I nurture myself with love and kindness,
drawing strength from the abundant love that surrounds me.

My strength, resilience, and spirit enable me to thrive.

Affirmations can be steady companions on your healing journey. When uncertainty arises, their words can offer love, courage, and a quiet confidence that you can navigate whatever comes your way. By practicing them, you will reconnect with your strength, your resilience, and your capacity to heal.

Afterword

"Faith is the bird that feels the light and
sings when the dawn is still dark."
—RABINDRANATH TAGORE, *Stray Birds*

This isn't just the end of the book—it's my last chance to connect with you.

As you step into the next phase of your journey, I want to offer encouragement and meet you where you are, especially if that place still feels raw or unfamiliar.

I remember those first weeks and months after my cancer diagnosis. It felt like being dropped into a foreign country with no map, no translator, and no time to catch my breath.

That's why I wrote this book—not because I had all the answers, but because I remember what it's like to need a companion. Someone to say, *I've been there. Here's what helped me. Maybe it will help you, too.*

This journey doesn't come with a clear road map. But maybe, through these pages, you've found something to hold onto—a way to steady yourself, meaningful questions to bring to your appointments, or a practice that helped you feel a little more like *you*. These tools are yours now. They'll be there when the path ahead feels uncertain.

Remember to take a deep breath. And when you're ready, step into what comes next—not with certainty, but with compassion, and trust in the care you've chosen.

As your healing continues to unfold, know that I am holding you in my thoughts—and quietly cheering you on.

—Jennifer

Financial Resources

"Asking for help isn't giving up.
It's refusing to give up."
—CHARLIE MACKESY, *The Boy, the Mole, the Fox and the Horse*

When I was newly diagnosed, I assumed the hardest part would be the medical treatment itself. I wasn't prepared for the flood of bills, insurance denials, and the crushing uncertainty about how we would manage the costs. I quickly learned that cancer doesn't just attack the body—it disrupts your finances, your sense of control, and your peace of mind.

If you're overwhelmed by the cost of care, you're not alone. The financial side of cancer is often one of the most under-discussed and most destabilizing parts of the journey. There is help. And there is hope.

This section is your tool kit: a collection of trusted organizations, practical tips, and insights to ease the burden and connect you with real, usable support. These resources exist because no one should have to choose between paying their bills and getting the treatment they need.

Whether you're just starting to navigate insurance or already juggling copays and out-of-pocket expenses, I hope these pages offer some relief so you can focus on what matters most.

The High Cost of Cancer Care

Cancer is one of the most expensive diseases to treat, second only to heart disease, according to the CDC.[1] The cost of care can vary greatly depending on the type and stage of your cancer, as well as the treatment plan recommended by your medical team. On average, cancer treatment can total around *$150,000*.[2] Some cancer drugs can cost over *$10,000 per month*, especially those used in targeted or advanced treatment plans. Patients often need a combination of these high-cost medications, ongoing specialized care, and coordination across multiple specialists to achieve the best possible outcome.

Cancer-related expenses typically fall into two categories: direct and indirect costs. Direct costs include surgery, chemotherapy, immunotherapy, radiation, and medications. Indirect costs may involve lost income, transportation, caregiving, and other out-of-pocket expenses.

Financial Toxicity: What It Is and How It Affects Your Care

Even with insurance, you may face significant out-of-pocket expenses that threaten your financial stability. The term "financial toxicity"—coined by Dr. S. Yousuf Zafar and Dr. Amy Abernethy of the Duke Cancer Institute—describes the burden of medical expenses that can diminish your quality of life and limit access to the care you deserve. For many, this means making painful trade-offs: skipping medications, delaying appointments, or choosing less effective treatments simply because of cost.

If you're underinsured or uninsured, you might have to drain your savings, take on debt, or even consider bankruptcy to continue treatment. And if you're working, the income you lose due to treatment-related absences can make things even harder. When you're already coping with the physical and emotional toll of cancer, these financial pressures can become overwhelming.

Mapping Out Your Financial Options

When you're navigating a cancer diagnosis, financial support isn't just helpful—it can be lifesaving. Patients who receive financial support have a 73 percent survival rate, compared to only 46 percent for those who don't.[3] That kind of difference speaks for itself—and underscores why seeking support early in your journey can make a real impact.

The good news is, you don't have to face the financial side of cancer alone. There are steps you can take and resources that can help. Once you have a diagnosis and a clearer picture of your treatment plan, it's important to assess the potential costs and begin exploring the support available to you. Many hospitals and cancer centers offer dedicated services to help ease the financial burden of care.

- **Talk to your oncologist about treatment costs.** While the best medical care should always be the priority, financial realities play a role in treatment decisions. It is your right to ask your doctor to consider the cost of care when discussing treatment options.

- **Meet with a financial counselor or social worker at your cancer center.** These professionals can help you understand your insurance, identify assistance programs, explore payment plans, and more.

- **Consider consulting a financial advisor.** Whether you need help budgeting for treatment or planning ahead, expert support can offer peace of mind and long-term stability.

Trusted Resources to Help You Navigate Costs

Below is a list of reliable resources that can make a real difference in covering the cost of care.

- **CancerCare's Financial Assistance Program**
  www.cancercare.org/financial_assistance
  CancerCare offers an online tool called *Helping Hand*—a searchable database with up-to-date contact information for financial and practical assistance from hundreds of national and regional organizations. You can search by diagnosis, zip code, and type of support to find resources tailored to your needs. Through CancerCare, you may also qualify for limited financial help with cancer-related costs such as transportation, home care, or childcare. If co-pays are a barrier, their programs can help cover the cost of prescribed treatments. Also, oncology social workers and co-payment specialists are available to connect you with additional support services and help identify resources that match your specific needs.

- **Family Reach**
  https://familyreach.org
  Family Reach is a national nonprofit that provides financial support to families facing cancer. Assistance may cover basic living expenses such as food, housing, utilities, and transportation.

- **TriageCancer.org**
  https://triagecancer.org
  Triage Cancer is a national nonprofit that helps individuals understand the legal and practical issues that can arise after a cancer diagnosis. Their resources cover topics like health insurance, employment rights, disability insurance, estate planning, and financial guidance. You can also access free educational events, downloadable materials, and a Legal & Financial Navigation Program, which supports patients, caregivers, and healthcare professionals alike.

- **MyHealthcareFinances**
  www.myhealthcarefinances.com
  MyHealthcareFinances is an online platform that provides clear, practical guidance to help you take control of your healthcare costs. You'll learn how insurance works, how to choose the right plan, and how to make the most of your coverage. The site also offers tools to help you manage medical bills, reduce costs before and after treatment, and find financial assistance. In addition, you'll gain insight into workplace protections, disability insurance options, and caregiver-specific resources and protections.

- **Good Days**
  https://mygooddays.org
  Good Days is a national nonprofit organization that provides financial assistance for those living with a chronic

or life-altering condition. Support may include help with copays, travel expenses, insurance premiums, and diagnostic testing.

Applicant requirements: To qualify, you must have a diagnosis that matches a condition currently covered by Good Days, and the program must be open for enrollment. You'll also need a valid Social Security number and must be receiving treatment in the United States. Your health insurance must cover at least 50 percent of your prescribed therapy, and your household income must be at or below 500 percent of the federal poverty level, based on your household size.

Nonprofit Programs for Copay Relief and Miscellaneous Expenses

- **CancerCare Co-Payment Assistance Foundation**
  www.cancercarecopay.org
  The CancerCare Co-Payment Assistance Foundation is a nonprofit organization dedicated to helping individuals overcome financial barriers to treatment by covering copayments for prescribed therapies. If copays for chemotherapy or targeted treatment drugs are keeping you from staying on track with your care, this program can help you access the treatment you need. Their streamlined enrollment process determines your eligibility right away, so you can begin receiving support without delay.

- **Blood Cancer United Co-Pay Assistance Program**
  https://bloodcancerunited.org/financial-assistance/co-pay-assistance-program
  The Co-Pay Assistance Program helps individuals with blood cancer offset the costs of private, Medicare, Medicaid, and

TRICARE (for members of the US military community) insurance premiums, as well as treatment-related co-pays and co-insurance for prescription drugs, labs, scans, and tests.

- **Patient Advocate Foundation (PAF) Co-Pay Relief Program**
  https://copays.org
  The Patient Advocate Foundation's Co-Pay Relief Program provides direct financial assistance to help cover copayments, coinsurance, and other cost-sharing expenses related to prescribed treatments and medications. Grants can also be used to help pay for your medical insurance premiums.

  Applicant requirements: To qualify for assistance, you must have a diagnosis that matches one of the specific disease funds currently supported by the program. You'll also need to meet the program's financial eligibility guidelines and have valid health insurance that covers the treatment or medication for which you're seeking help.

- **HealthWell Foundation**
  www.healthwellfoundation.org
  The HealthWell Foundation is an independent nonprofit organization that helps reduce the financial burden of care for individuals who are underinsured and living with chronic or life-altering illnesses. Since 2004, they've awarded grants to more than 1.1 million people. In 2024 alone, they provided over $1.2 billion in assistance through their Disease Funds. If you qualify, the HealthWell Foundation may help you cover a range of out-of-pocket expenses, including coinsurance and copayments for prescription medications, monthly health insurance premiums, deductibles, and other medical-related costs such as surgeries, supplies, or supplements.

  Applicant requirements: To qualify for assistance, you must have some form of health insurance. This includes private insurance, Medicare, Medicaid, or Tricare. You also need to be diagnosed with a condition covered by one of HealthWell's Disease Funds; you can check their website to see which funds are currently open. Your household income should fall within 300 percent to 500 percent of the federal poverty level, adjusted for the cost of living in your area. Additionally, you must be receiving treatment in the United States, as the foundation only supports care delivered within the country.

- **The Pink Fund**
  https://pinkfund.org
  If you're undergoing active treatment for breast cancer, the Pink Fund may be able to help. They offer short-term financial assistance to cover essential nonmedical living expenses, such as housing, transportation, utilities, and insurance, so you can focus on your health without added financial stress.

- **National Organization for Rare Disorders (NORD)**
  https://rarediseases.org
  NORD is a nonprofit organization that offers financial assistance, advocacy, and resources for people living with rare diseases, including rare cancers. Through their patient assistance programs, they can help you access treatment, join clinical trials, and connect with specialized care providers.

- **Accessia Health**
  https://accessiahealth.org
  Accessia Health provides support for insurance premiums, medication copayments, travel, and other essential medical expenses if you have a qualifying chronic condition and meet their household income requirements, regardless of your age.

- **The SAMFund (a program of Expect Miracles Foundation)**
  https://expectmiraclesfoundation.org/samfund
  The SAMFund offers grants to young adult cancer survivors, helping with essential expenses such as medical bills, rent or mortgage payments, tuition, student loans, and transportation. The program also supports fertility preservation, recognizing its critical role at this stage of life.

- **Modest Needs Foundation**
  www.modestneeds.org
  Modest Needs provides short-term financial assistance for individuals working and earning just above the poverty line—often too much to qualify for traditional aid, yet not enough to cover unexpected expenses. Their grants can help you stay self-sufficient and avoid falling into long-term financial hardship.

- **Cancer Financial Assistance Coalition (CFAC)**
  www.cancerfac.org
  CFAC is a coalition of national organizations working together to help you manage the financial challenges associated with cancer. They connect you to resources, educate you and your care team about available support, and advocate on your behalf to help reduce the financial burdens of treatment. You can also search their online database to find financial assistance programs by diagnosis, treatment type, or specific need.

- **Mission4Maureen**
  https://mission4maureen.org
  Mission4Maureen is a nonprofit organization that offers financial assistance to individuals diagnosed with brain cancer or a brain tumor. They may be able to help with rent, mortgage payments, utilities, medical bills, and other daily

living costs, easing the financial burden that often comes with treatment.

Pharmaceutical Patient Assistance Programs

Many pharmaceutical companies offer patient assistance programs to help cover the cost of expensive medications, particularly for individuals who are uninsured or underinsured. To find out if you're eligible, contact the manufacturer directly and ask to speak with customer service or the patient assistance department.

▶ Nonprofit Programs for Prescription Assistance

- **NeedyMeds**
  https://needymeds.org
  NeedyMeds is a national nonprofit that helps you find free or low-cost options for prescriptions and other healthcare expenses. Through its website, you can search for patient assistance programs for pharmaceuticals, locate free or sliding-scale clinics across the country, and access a wide range of coupons and rebates. NeedyMeds also offers a free drug discount card that can significantly lower the cost of medications at many pharmacies nationwide. All of these tools are available online—no registration required.

- **Patient Access Network Foundation (PAN Foundation)**
  www.panfoundation.org
  The PAN Foundation is a nonprofit that helps cover out-of-pocket costs for prescribed medications if you're underinsured. If you're living with a serious or chronic illness, PAN offers grants and support programs to help you access the treatments you need.

- **RxAssist**
  www.rxassist.org
  You can search this comprehensive online database to find pharmaceutical company programs that offer free or low-cost medications if you're unable to afford your prescriptions.

- **RxHope**
  www.rxhope.com
  RxHope is a national online resource that helps you access medications you may not be able to afford. It advocates on your behalf, simplifying the patient assistance process by offering vital information and support. You can search by medication to find Patient Assistance Programs (PAPs) that offer free or low-cost prescriptions. In many cases, your provider can apply on your behalf, and no patient account is required to explore available programs.

- **Rx Outreach**
  https://rxoutreach.org
  Rx Outreach is a nonprofit mail-order pharmacy that helps individuals and families access affordable prescription medications, especially if they're uninsured or underinsured. You may qualify if your household income is at or below 400 percent of the federal poverty level, even if you have Medicare, Medicaid, or another insurance plan.

A Public-Benefit Pharmacy for Affordable Medications

- **CostPlus Drugs**
  www.costplusdrugs.com
  Founded by Mark Cuban, CostPlus Drugs is a public-benefit, for-profit mail-order pharmacy serving the general public. (A public-benefit corporation is a for-profit company that

commits to serving a social good as part of its legal mission.) It reduces drug costs through transparent pricing and minimal markup, cutting out middlemen. You can browse available medications and place orders directly through the website—no insurance required. While it doesn't currently accept insurance, its listed prices are often lower than typical copays.

▶ Prescription Discount Programs

- **Drug Discount Cards**

  Some states, nonprofit organizations, and retail pharmacies offer drug discount cards. A few are free, while others charge a low monthly or annual fee. If you're paying for one, make sure it's through a reputable source, such as AARP or NeedyMeds.

  Warning: Scammers sometimes sell fake discount cards to steal credit card or Social Security numbers. Be aware that discount cards are *not* health insurance. Before signing up, review the terms and conditions carefully and make sure the card includes at least a thirty-day refund policy.

Government Assistance

Several federal and state programs offer financial benefits to individuals and families. These benefits—often referred to as *entitlements*—are typically intended for low-income individuals, seniors, and people with disabilities. Each program has its own eligibility requirements, and availability may vary depending on where you live and current legislation. Given the changing political landscape, some programs may be expanded, reduced, or restructured in the future. It's important to stay informed and check for the most up-to-date information, especially when applying. Depending on your situation, you may also qualify for additional state-based programs that can help with health-care-related costs.

Government assistance programs include:

- **US Department of Health & Human Services**
  www.hhs.gov
  You may qualify for help through programs like Medicaid, Medicare, and the Health Resources and Services Administration (HRSA), which offer coverage for medical care, prescription assistance, and certain forms of financial support for people with low incomes.

- **Centers for Medicare & Medicaid Services (CMS)**
  www.cms.gov
  Please note that Medicaid does not have a single national customer service line like Medicare, as it is managed at the state level. Each state has its own Medicaid office with a dedicated customer service number.

- **US Administration for Community Living Eldercare Locator**
  https://eldercare.acl.gov
  The Eldercare Locator is a nationwide service that can connect you or an older loved one with trustworthy local support resources. These may include transportation, in-home services, meal delivery, caregiver support, housing assistance, and help navigating Medicare and other benefits.

- **Social Security Administration (SSA)**
  www.ssa.gov
  If you're unable to work due to cancer, the SSA offers financial assistance through two main programs. Social Security Disability Insurance (SSDI) provides monthly benefits if you've worked and paid into Social Security and your disability prevents you from working. Supplemental Security Income (SSI)

offers monthly financial support if you have limited income and resources and haven't paid into Social Security.

The SSA also has a Compassionate Allowances (CAL) program that speeds up the application review process for individuals with serious medical conditions, including certain aggressive or advanced-stage cancers, enabling quicker access to benefits. To learn more or apply, visit www.ssa.gov/compassionateallowances or contact your local Social Security office.

Free and Low-Cost Transportation for Local and Remote Care

If you need to travel a long distance for specialized treatment—or face transportation barriers close to home—you're not alone. For those who are immunocompromised, commercial travel can feel risky or financially out of reach. Fortunately, several organizations offer support. Some match patients with volunteer pilots who donate their time and aircraft, while others provide access to unused seats on corporate or private jets. These programs are designed to help you reach the care you need, whether it's across town or across the country.

- **American Cancer Society Road To Recovery Program**
  www.cancer.org/support-programs-and-services/road-to-recovery.html
  Trained volunteers can drive you or a family member to and from hospitals or clinics for treatment. Call the American Cancer Society to see if the Road To Recovery program is currently available in your area.

- **Air Care Alliance (ACA)**
  www.aircarealliance.org

The ACA connects individuals with volunteer pilot organizations (VPOs) across the United States that offer free air transportation for medical and humanitarian needs. While ACA does not arrange flights directly, it serves as a central hub to help you access the right organization for your needs. You can submit a flight request through their website and will be referred to a VPO that best fits your situation.

Applicant requirements: Each VPO sets its own eligibility criteria, but most require that you demonstrate financial need, be medically stable, and have a verifiable medical reason for travel—usually confirmed by a physician's medical release. You must also be able to enter and exit a small aircraft with minimal assistance (this may involve climbing steps or stepping onto a wing) and be able to sit upright with a seatbelt fastened throughout the flight.

Advance notice requirements: At least two weeks

- **Air Charity Network**
  https://aircharitynetwork.org
  This organization is a network of regional member groups that coordinate free volunteer pilot flights across the continental United States, as well as Alaska and Hawaii.

  Applicant requirements: To qualify, you must demonstrate a financial or physical need. All adult passengers must be able to walk unassisted. Most of the aircraft used are small, unpressurized planes with four to six seats. Getting in and out is similar to climbing into and out of the back seat of a compact car. You must also be able to sit upright and wear a seatbelt for the entire flight.

  Advance notice requirements: At least two weeks

- **Angel Flight West (AFW)**
  https://angelflightwest.org
  Angel Flight West provides free air transportation to medical

appointments for residents of the following twelve western states: Alaska, Arizona, California, Colorado, Hawaii, Idaho, Nevada, Montana, Oregon, Utah, Washington, and Wyoming. Volunteer pilots donate their time and cover the cost of each flight, which typically ranges from one hundred to nine hundred miles.

Applicant requirements: To qualify, you must demonstrate a financial, medical, or geographic need. You should be able to walk independently, get in and out of a small plane without assistance, and remain seated upright with a seatbelt fastened for the entire flight. Travel must be tied to a scheduled medical appointment or procedure, and your healthcare provider will need to complete a form confirming you're fit to fly.

Advance notice requirements: At least seven days

- **Corporate Angel Network (CAN)**
  www.corpangelnetwork.org
  You may be eligible for flight assistance through Corporate Angel Network, which arranges free travel for cancer patients by filling empty seats on corporate and private jets donated by businesses and individuals.

  Applicant requirements: To qualify, you must be able to walk up the steps of a corporate aircraft without assistance and cannot require oxygen, IV medications, or medical support during the flight. Flights are available to all active cancer patients, as well as bone marrow and stem cell donors and recipients. Financial need is not required, and there's no limit to how often you can fly.

  Advance notice requirements: Submit a flight request up to ten business days before your scheduled travel.

- **Mercy Medical Angels**
  www.mercymedical.org

Mercy Medical Angels offers several types of transportation assistance for eligible individuals. You may receive free commercial airline tickets for yourself and a medically necessary escort to travel anywhere in the United States. You may qualify for free flights with volunteer pilots if you're able to walk on your own and don't need medical care during the trip. Mercy Medical Angels also provides ground transportation support such as gas cards, bus tickets, and train fare to help you reach your medical appointments. The organization operates multiple programs to support patients and veterans alike.

Applicant requirements: To qualify for assistance, you must demonstrate financial need by providing income verification, including total household income and assets. You must also be able to walk independently, get in and out of a plane with little or no help, and travel without requiring medical support.

Advance notice requirements: To ensure your request can be processed in time, you'll need to plan ahead. For commercial airline tickets, apply at least twenty-one days before your travel date. If you need help with ground transportation (gas/bus/train), apply at least fourteen business days in advance. For volunteer pilot flights, be sure to submit your request at least ten days before your intended travel.

- **Miracle Flights**
  https://miracleflights.org
  If your child needs medical care that isn't available in your local community, Miracle Flights may be able to help. This national nonprofit provides free commercial airline tickets for children and their families, allowing you to travel anywhere in the United States as often as needed for essential treatment.

  Applicant requirements: To qualify, your child must be seventeen or younger and medically cleared to fly on a commercial airline. You must have a confirmed medical appointment that requires air travel, verified by the treatment site. Up to two parents or legal guardians may accompany your child on each flight. Your family's gross income must generally be at or below three times the federal poverty guidelines, based on household size.

Advance notice requirements: Flight request applications, treatment site verification forms, and supporting documentation should be submitted at least fourteen days before the requested departure date to allow time to coordinate your flight.

Free and Low-Cost Lodging

If you need to travel for medical care, you and your caregiver may have to be away from home for weeks or even months. While this can be a costly experience, there are resources that offer rooms, suites, or even entire homes at little or no cost.

- **American Cancer Society (ACS)**
  www.cancer.org
  The American Cancer Society offers lodging programs to help you and your loved ones stay close to care during cancer treatment.

  Through its flagship Hope Lodge program, you and a caregiver can stay for free at one of more than thirty locations across the United States and Puerto Rico while you're undergoing active cancer treatment.

  You may also be eligible for discounted hotel accommodations through ACS's partnership with Extended Stay America, which includes over seven hundred locations nationwide. Eligibility and rates for this program are determined by ACS based on financial need.

  There is no strict limit to the length of your stay; how long you can remain depends on your treatment plan and room availability. All Hope Lodge accommodations are free of charge. For Extended Stay America, ACS will evaluate your financial need to determine eligibility for free or reduced-rate lodging.

Applicant requirements: To stay at Hope Lodge, you must be in active cancer treatment, live more than forty miles or one hour from your treatment center, and be accompanied by a caregiver.

Note: Because lodging programs and partnerships may change, visit the ACS website or call their toll-free number for the most up-to-date information.

- **Joe's House**

  www.joeshouse.org

  Joe's House is a nonprofit founded by Ann Calahan in memory of her husband, Joe. If you're looking for a place to stay during treatment, Joe's House is an excellent online resource that lists thousands of lodging options near hospitals and treatment centers across the country. You'll find everything from discounted hotel stays—offered in partnership with national chains—to nonprofit housing, motels, apartments, home-sharing programs, and even RV parks. It's designed to help you and your loved ones find affordable, comfortable lodging during a challenging time. Your length of stay will depend on your treatment schedule and the policies of the lodging facility. There's no fixed limit; it's based on your needs and availability. Pricing can range from free (nonprofit housing) to between 10 percent and 25 percent off the best available rates at the time of booking. Discounts vary depending on the lodging partner and location.

  Applicant requirements: Eligibility requirements vary by lodging facility. While Joe's House primarily serves people with cancer, many of the listed options also welcome patients with other medical conditions.

- **Healthcare Hospitality Network (HHN)**
  www.hhnetwork.org
  HHN is a nationwide network of more than two hundred nonprofit organizations that provide you and your family with free or deeply discounted lodging while you're receiving medical care far from home. The length of your stay at an HHN member facility will depend on your treatment plan and the specific house. Some offer short stays of just a few days, while others accommodate longer visits lasting several weeks or even months. Each healthcare hospitality house sets its own rates, but lodging is typically free or offered at a significantly reduced cost.

  Applicant requirements: Each hospital's hospitality house has its own eligibility criteria.

- **Ronald McDonald House Charities (RMHC)**
  https://rmhc.org
  RMHC operates over 385 Houses worldwide, along with Family Rooms and Care Mobiles. These Houses offer families a place to stay close to the hospital when a child requires medical treatment, with meals, bedrooms, and common spaces. Referrals usually come through a hospital social worker or care team. Some locations may have waiting lists. While a donation may be suggested, many stays are free, and no family is turned away for inability to pay. To get started, ask your hospital's social services department about the RMHC program in your area.

  Applicant requirements: Generally, you can stay at a Ronald McDonald House if your child receiving treatment is twenty-one years old or younger. However, because of high demand, some locations may limit accommodations to families of patients up to age eighteen.

- **Fisher House Foundation**
  https://fisherhouse.org
  Fisher House Foundation builds homes where military and veterans' families can stay free of charge while a loved one is hospitalized. Located at military and VA medical centers around the world, these homes provide comfortable lodging for as long as it's needed. Families are welcome to stay as long as their loved one is receiving care, with no cost ever required.

  Applicant requirements: Patient selection criteria are determined by the commander or director of each medical center where the Fisher House is located.

Patient Advocacy and Financial Assistance

- **Patient Advocate Foundation (PAF)**
  www.patientadvocate.org
  PAF is a national nonprofit organization established in 1996 that provides professional case management services and financial aid to Americans with chronic, life-threatening, and debilitating illnesses. Services include one-on-one case management to help you resolve healthcare access issues, insurance denials, and medical debt crises. If you're insured and meet certain qualifications, the Co-Pay Relief Program may offer direct financial assistance for prescriptions and treatments. Additionally, you may qualify for a small grant through PAF's Financial Aid Funds to cover nonmedical expenses that could interfere with your treatment.

  PAF also offers a wide range of educational resources, legal counseling, and referrals to help you navigate managed care, insurance challenges, financial concerns, job discrimination, and debt.

Free Financial Planning Services

- **Pro Bono Financial Planners**
  https://familyreach.org
  https://ffpprobono.org
  www.financialplanningassociation.org
  The Financial Planning for Cancer program connects you with a pro bono financial planner to help manage cash flow, debt, and other financial challenges during treatment. The program is a collaboration between Family Reach, the Foundation for Financial Planning (FFP), and the Financial Planning Association (FPA). To get started, reach out to any of the listed organizations.

Glossary

benign. In the context of cancer, benign refers to a tumor or growth that is noncancerous. Benign tumors do not invade nearby tissues or spread to other parts of the body (metastasize). They are typically less harmful than malignant (cancerous) tumors, but they can still cause problems if they press on vital organs or structures.

biomarker. A biomarker (short for biological marker) is a measurable substance, characteristic, or molecule found in the body that provides information about normal biological processes, disease conditions, or responses to treatment. Biomarkers can be found in blood, tissues, urine, or other body fluids, and are used in diagnosing, monitoring, and treating various diseases, including cancer.

biomarker testing. Biomarker testing (also called molecular testing, genomic testing, or tumor profiling) is a laboratory process used to analyze a patient's blood, tissue, or other body fluids for specific biomarkers—molecules that provide information about a disease. In cancer care, biomarker testing helps identify genetic mutations, proteins, or other cellular changes that influence tumor growth and response to treatment. It is a key component of precision medicine—cancer treatments tailored to a patient's unique tumor profile rather than a one-size-fits-all approach.

biopsy. A medical procedure in which a small sample of cells or tissue is removed from the body for examination under a microscope. Biopsies are used to determine whether cancer or other abnormal cells are present and can help identify the type, grade, and extent of a disease. They are often performed when imaging or physical exams reveal a suspicious area.

BRCA (pronounced BRAH-kuh or B-R-C-A). Stands for "BReast CAncer" gene. Mutations in BRCA1 or BRCA2 significantly increase the risk of breast and ovarian cancers. These risks underscore the importance of genetic testing, risk assessment, and counseling for individuals with a family history of BRCA-related cancers.

chemo brain. A term used to describe cognitive impairments, such as memory lapses, difficulty concentrating, and trouble multitasking, that may occur during or after cancer treatment, especially chemotherapy.

chemotherapy. A type of cancer treatment that uses powerful chemical (chemo) drugs to destroy cancer cells.

clinical trial. A research study with human participants that tests the safety and effectiveness of a medical treatment, procedure, drug, or device. These studies follow strict rules to protect participants and increase the reliability of results.

complementary therapy. Nonmedical treatments used alongside conventional cancer care to support physical, emotional, or spiritual well-being. Examples discussed in this book include meditation, guided imagery, somatic yoga, Jin Shin Jyutsu,

Qigong, Feldenkrais, and Reiki. These therapies are not intended to replace medical treatment but may help ease symptoms, reduce stress, and improve quality of life.

CT scan (computed tomography). An advanced imaging test that uses a series of X-rays taken from different angles to create detailed cross-sectional images of internal structures, such as bones, organs, and blood vessels. These images are processed by a computer to provide a three-dimensional view of the body. CT scans are commonly used to detect tumors or abnormalities, diagnose conditions, guide treatments, and monitor progress.

electronic health record (EHR). A digital version of a patient's medical history, accessible to authorized healthcare providers and, often, to patients themselves through a secure online portal.

explanation of benefits (EOB). A statement provided by a health insurance company to its policyholder after a medical service has been processed. The EOB outlines the details of the claim, including the services received, the cost of those services, any discounts or adjustments, what the insurance covers, and the remaining balance the patient may owe. It is not a bill but a summary of how the claim was handled, including the patient's financial responsibility, if any.

Feldenkrais (pronounced FELL-den-krice). A therapeutic approach that uses gentle, mindful movements and focused awareness to improve physical function, enhance mobility, and relieve tension. Developed by Dr. Moshe Feldenkrais in the 1940s, this method is based on the understanding that habitual movement patterns and postures can contribute to discomfort, pain, or limited physical ability. It is widely used in rehabilitation, pain management, and performance improvement in sports, music, and dance.

genetic. Relating to genes and heredity. In cancer care, the term is often used in the context of risk assessment, as certain inherited genetic mutations (such as BRCA1 and BRCA2) can increase a person's likelihood of developing specific cancers.

genetic counselor. A healthcare professional trained in genetics and counseling who helps individuals understand their risk for inherited conditions, such as cancer. Genetic counselors assess hereditary risk, explain test results, and guide patients in understanding the implications for themselves and their families. This information can significantly influence treatment decisions, including choices about surgery, targeted therapies, and long-term monitoring for potential health issues.

genetic testing. A medical test that analyzes DNA to identify changes or mutations in genes. It is often used to assess a person's risk of developing certain inherited conditions, including cancer.

guided imagery. A therapeutic relaxation technique that involves the use of mental visualization to create calming and positive sensory experiences. Often used as a complementary therapy, guided imagery is considered beneficial for managing anxiety, alleviating pain, improving sleep, and supporting overall mental health.

hormone therapy. Treatment that removes, blocks, or adds hormones to slow or stop the growth of hormone-sensitive cancers.

immunotherapy. A type of cancer treatment that helps the body's immune system recognize, attack, and destroy cancer cells. Unlike traditional treatments like chemotherapy or radiation, which often affect both cancerous and healthy cells, immunotherapy boosts the body's natural defenses to specifically target and fight cancer more effectively.

integrative oncologist. A medical doctor specializing in cancer treatment who combines conventional therapies, such as surgery, chemotherapy, radiation, and immunotherapy, with evidence-based complementary approaches to support overall well-being. These integrative approaches are designed to ease treatment side effects and strengthen the mind-body connection. By supporting physical, emotional, and spiritual health, they can improve resilience and quality of life during and after treatment. Integrative oncologists work collaboratively with both conventional medical teams and complementary care providers to create personalized treatment plans grounded in scientific evidence and individual preferences.

integrative oncology. A patient-centered approach to cancer care that combines conventional medical treatments, such as surgery, chemotherapy, radiation, and immunotherapy, with evidence-based complementary therapies. The goal is to treat the whole person, not just the disease. Integrative oncology supports physical, emotional, and spiritual well-being by easing side effects, enhancing quality of life, and strengthening resilience throughout the cancer journey. Care is delivered by a coordinated team that may include both conventional and complementary providers, working together to align treatment with the patient's values, needs, and preferences.

Jin Shin Jyutsu (pronounced Jin-SHIN-Jit-Soo). An ancient Japanese healing art that seeks to harmonize the body's energy pathways (meridians) to promote physical, emotional, and spiritual well-being. The practice involves gentle touch and specific hand placements on designated points or "safety energy locks" located throughout the body. These points are believed to correspond to areas where energy may become blocked or stagnant. By applying focused touch, practitioners or individuals aim to restore the natural flow of energy, supporting the body's innate ability to heal itself. Jin Shin Jyutsu is used to reduce stress, alleviate pain, improve circulation, and enhance overall vitality.

leukemia. A type of cancer that affects the blood and bone marrow.

lumpectomy. A surgery to remove a tumor from the breast while preserving most of the breast tissue.

lymph nodes. Small, bean-shaped structures that are part of the lymphatic system. Lymph nodes filter lymph fluid, trapping bacteria, viruses, and cancer cells to help the immune system fight infections and other diseases. They are found throughout the body, including the neck, armpits, chest, abdomen, and groin. Swollen or enlarged lymph nodes can sometimes indicate infection, inflammation, or the spread of cancer.

lymphatic system. A vital part of the immune system that helps protect the body from infection and disease. It includes a network of lymph vessels, lymph nodes, and organs—such as the spleen, thymus, and tonsils—that circulate lymph, a fluid containing white blood cells, throughout the body. The lymphatic system helps remove waste, toxins, and excess fluids, and plays a key role in identifying and fighting infections and abnormal cells, including cancer.

lymphedema. A condition in which excess lymph fluid builds up in the tissues, causing swelling—most commonly in the arms or legs. It often occurs when the lymphatic system is damaged or blocked, typically following cancer treatment such as surgery, radiation, or lymph node removal. Lymphedema can be managed through approaches like compression garments, gentle exercise, massage, and specialized physical therapy.

malignant. Refers to a tumor or growth that is cancerous and can invade nearby tissues and spread (metastasize) to other parts of the body. Malignant tumors grow aggressively and can pose a serious threat to health if not treated.

mammogram. A specialized X-ray imaging test used to examine breast tissue. It plays a key role in the early detection and diagnosis of breast cancer by revealing abnormalities, such as lumps, calcifications, or distortions, often before they can be felt during a physical exam.

mastectomy. A surgery to remove one or both breasts, typically to treat or prevent cancer.

medical oncology. The branch of oncology focused on treating cancer using medications such as chemotherapy, immunotherapy, hormone therapy, and targeted therapy.

metastatic. Refers to cancer that has spread from its original location (primary site) to other parts of the body, forming new tumors in organs, tissues, or lymph nodes.

metastatic cancer. Also known as stage 4 cancer, metastatic cancer is more difficult to treat because it involves multiple areas of the body.

Mindfulness-Based Stress Reduction (MBSR). An evidence-based program developed by Dr. Jon Kabat-Zinn that combines mindfulness meditation, body awareness, and gentle yoga to help individuals reduce stress and improve physical and emotional well-being. Originally designed to support patients with chronic pain and stress-related conditions, MBSR teaches participants how to cultivate present-moment awareness and develop a nonjudgmental attitude toward their experiences. It is widely used in healthcare and wellness settings to support mental health, manage chronic illness, and enhance overall quality of life.

MRI (magnetic resonance imaging). A noninvasive medical imaging technique that uses powerful magnets, radio waves, and a computer to create detailed images of organs, soft tissues, and other internal structures—without using radiation. It is especially useful for detecting abnormalities in the brain, spine, joints, and internal organs, and is often used in cancer care to evaluate tumors, monitor treatment progress, and guide surgical planning.

multidisciplinary team. A group of healthcare professionals from different specialties who collaborate to develop a patient's treatment plan.

oncologist. A doctor who specializes in diagnosing and treating cancer.

oncology. The study and treatment of cancer.

palliative care (pronounced PAL-ee-uh-tiv care). Specialized medical care focused on improving the quality of life for individuals with serious or chronic illnesses. It addresses physical, emotional, psychological, and spiritual needs to relieve symptoms such as pain, fatigue, shortness of breath, or stress. Palliative care can be provided alongside curative treatments or as the primary focus of care, depending on the individual's goals and condition. It is available at any stage of a serious illness and is distinct from hospice care, which specifically focuses on end-of-life care.

pathology report. A detailed medical document that provides information about a diagnosis based on the examination of tissue, cells, or bodily fluids removed during a biopsy or surgery. Prepared by a pathologist, the report contains critical details about the sample, such as whether it is benign or malignant, the type and stage of cancer (if present), and other characteristics that help guide treatment decisions.

PET scan (positron emission tomography). An imaging test that uses a small amount of radioactive material (called a radiotracer) to create detailed images of how tissues and organs function in the body. Unlike CT or MRI scans, which focus on structural details, a PET scan highlights metabolic activity at the cellular level. It is used to detect cancer cells because they typically have a higher metabolic rate than normal cells. During a PET scan, the radiotracer (often a form of glucose labeled with a radioactive atom) is absorbed more by cancer cells, as they consume glucose at a faster rate. This allows the PET scan to detect areas of abnormal activity, making it particularly useful for detecting cancer, staging cancer, monitoring treatment, and identifying recurrence.

prebiotics. Nondigestible fibers that nourish beneficial bacteria in the gut, promoting digestive health.

precision medicine. Precision medicine, also known as personalized medicine, is an approach that tailors medical treatment to an individual's unique genetic, molecular, environmental, and lifestyle factors. Instead of using a one-size-fits-all strategy, it analyzes specific characteristics, such as biomarkers, genetic mutations, and tumor profiles, to determine the most effective treatments for a particular patient. This approach increases treatment effectiveness, improves survival rates, and minimizes side effects by ensuring that patients receive the right treatment at the right time.

probiotics. Live beneficial bacteria that support gut health and may improve digestion and immune function.

prognosis. The likely course or expected outcome of a disease, including chances of recovery, recurrence, or survival. It is based on factors such as the type and stage of the disease, the patient's overall health, and how well the condition is likely to respond to treatment.

protocol. A standardized plan or set of guidelines for medical treatment. Protocols outline the specific procedures, medications, dosages, and timing used to treat a particular condition, and are often based on clinical research or expert consensus to ensure consistency, safety, and effectiveness in patient care.

Qigong (pronounced chee-GONG). A traditional Chinese practice rooted in ancient medicine, martial arts, and philosophy. It integrates coordinated body movements, focused breathing techniques, and meditative states to cultivate and balance chi, which is believed to be the vital energy that flows through the body. Qigong aims to improve physical health, enhance mental clarity, and promote emotional balance. It is often used as a holistic approach to wellness and is practiced in various forms, ranging from gentle, slow movements to more dynamic routines. Qigong is also used in traditional Chinese medicine as a complementary therapy to support healing, reduce stress, and strengthen the body's resilience against illness.

radiation oncology. The medical specialty that uses high-energy radiation to treat cancer by shrinking or destroying tumors while aiming to minimize damage to surrounding healthy tissue.

radiation therapy. The use of high-energy radiation to kill cancer cells and shrink tumors.

radiologist. A medical doctor who specializes in interpreting medical imaging, such as X-rays, MRIs, CT scans, and ultrasounds, to diagnose disease.

Reiki (pronounced RAY-kee). A Japanese energy healing practice that can be done by a practitioner or by the individual. It uses gentle touch or hands hovering above the body to channel energy. By tapping into universal life force energy, Reiki aims to stimulate the body's natural healing response. This energy is believed to promote relaxation, reduce stress, and restore physical, emotional, and spiritual balance. Reiki is often used as a complementary therapy in integrative healthcare settings to support patients undergoing medical treatment.

sentinel lymph node biopsy (SLNB). A procedure used to identify and remove the sentinel node(s) to check for cancer cells. If no cancer is found, it is unlikely that cancer has spread, potentially reducing the need for more extensive lymph node removal. The results of a sentinel node biopsy help doctors determine the most appropriate treatment, including surgery, radiation, and chemotherapy. This technique is commonly used in breast cancer and melanoma but can be applied to other cancers as well.

sentinel node. The first lymph node (or group of nodes) to which cancer cells are most likely to spread from a primary tumor. Because lymph fluid drains from the tumor area into the sentinel node(s) first, testing these nodes can help determine whether cancer has spread beyond its original location.

somatic yoga. A gentle, mindful practice that combines traditional yoga poses and movements with techniques that promote heightened body awareness and the release of tension. Rooted in the principles of somatics, which emphasize the connection between mind and body, somatic yoga encourages practitioners to focus inward, exploring how their body feels during movement. This practice often involves slow, deliberate movements, breathwork, and mindful pauses to enhance relaxation, improve mobility, and reduce stress. It is particularly beneficial for individuals recovering from injury, managing chronic pain, or seeking to cultivate a deeper sense of connection with their physical and emotional well-being.

staging. The process of determining how much cancer is in the body and how far it has spread. Staging helps guide treatment decisions and estimate prognosis. Most cancers are staged from 0 to 4, with higher numbers indicating more advanced disease.

surgical oncology. The medical specialty focused on the surgical removal of tumors and cancerous tissue as part of cancer treatment.

targeted therapy. A cancer treatment that targets specific genes or proteins involved in cancer growth.

telemedicine. Remote medical consultations and treatment using digital communication technology. Often used to expand access to care—especially for patients in rural or underserved communities.

tumor. A mass or lump formed by an abnormal growth of cells. Tumors can be benign (noncancerous), meaning they don't spread to other parts of the body, or malignant (cancerous), meaning they can invade nearby tissues and potentially spread to distant organs.

ultrasound. A noninvasive imaging technique that uses high-frequency sound waves to create real-time images of the inside of the body. In cancer care, ultrasound is often used to detect tumors, guide biopsies, monitor treatment response, or evaluate organs for signs of cancer spread. Unlike imaging methods that use radiation, ultrasound is considered safe and is especially useful for examining soft tissues and fluid-filled areas.

X-ray. A quick, noninvasive imaging test that uses a small amount of electromagnetic radiation to produce images of the inside of the body. X-rays are especially effective for visualizing bones, certain organs, and abnormal growths, as different tissues absorb radiation at varying levels. They can help detect tumors or masses in areas like the lungs, bones, or breasts (as in a mammogram). X-rays can also distinguish between solid and fluid-filled growths, which may offer insight into whether a mass is likely to be benign or malignant. They are often used to track changes in tumors, assess cancer spread to bones, and guide instruments during procedures such as biopsies. While highly valuable in cancer care, X-rays involve a small dose of radiation and are used judiciously to balance the benefits of diagnosis with patient safety.

Acknowledgments

Writing *Just Diagnosed* has been one of the most personal and meaningful journeys of my life. I could not have completed it without the generous support, encouragement, and wisdom of so many extraordinary people.

To Debu Tripathy, MD: Thank you for lending your voice to the foreword. Your pioneering work in breast cancer research—particularly in the development of targeted therapies and personalized medicine—and your generous belief in this project brought both credibility and heart to these pages.

To the integrative and medical specialists who shared your time, knowledge, and insights: Thank you for shaping not only this book, but also the way I live my life. I'm especially grateful to Natalie Ledesma, JeanMarie Murphy, Jill Pasquinelli, Lonner Holden, Shirley Dockstader, and Kathleen Golden for your contributions to my chapters on nutrition, somatic yoga, Jin Shin Jyutsu, Qigong, and Reiki. Your presence in my healing journey is woven throughout these pages.

To Alan Newman, MD, my former oncologist at California Pacific Medical Center in San Francisco: Thank you for your knowledge, wisdom, and compassion, which always made me feel seen, heard, and deeply supported.

To the publishing team at She Writes Press: Thank you for believing in this book and bringing it to life with such care. Your guidance and partnership have meant the world to me.

To Margie Levine, mentor, cancer coach, and author of *Surviving Cancer*: You were both a guide and an inspiration. Though you're no longer with us, your strength and spirit live on in these pages and in everyone you've touched.

To Lidia Schapira, MD, fellow of the American Society of Clinical Oncology and director of cancer survivorship at Stanford Medicine, for generously sharing your insights on patient navigators and the vital role they play in the cancer journey.

To my writing mentors, critique partners, and early readers—especially those who sat with these pages while they were still finding their footing: Thank you for your thoughtful feedback and for believing in my vision before it fully took shape.

To Deborah Todd, my editor and dear friend: From the earliest days of my diagnosis, you've been a calm and trusted voice—guiding, shaping, and holding space for this book to become what it needed to be. Your belief in me gave me the courage to keep writing.

To my husband, Ty: Your quiet strength and unwavering love have carried me through the hardest moments of my life. You've stood by me with such tenderness, believing in me—and in this book—from the very beginning. And your brilliant sense of humor, even in the darkest times, has made it so much easier for me to laugh, breathe, and keep going. I couldn't have made it through without you.

To my son, Zac: Your arrival, just sixteen months before my diagnosis, awakened in me a fierce will to survive. I've watched you grow into someone whose deep empathy and compassion reflect the path we've traveled together.

To my family and friends—my father, Ray; my sister, Karen; my brother, Clark; and my dear friends Jean Ray, Kathy Levinsky, Robin Andrews, Katy Evelyn, and Divina Infusino: Thank you for the many hours you spent reading, listening, and reflecting as these pages unfolded. Your collective wisdom helped shape the heart of this book. It would not be the same without you.

And to Aristaeus, my Maine Coon companion: Thank you for reminding me, daily, to stretch, breathe, and pause. You were my fuzzy thread of calm through it all.

Finally, to the newly diagnosed reader: This book was written for you. If it brings you greater clarity, strength, or hope—even just a little—I'll know it has done its job.

Notes

CHAPTER 1: TAKE A DEEP BREATH

1. W. Dhillon, N. Abd Al-Noor, A. Gill, N. Gupta, V. DeBari, G. Guron, et al., "Impact of Deep Breathing and Relaxation Exercises on Health-Related Quality of Life in Breast Cancer Patients Receiving Chemotherapy," *Cancer Research* 69, no. 24_Supplement (2009): 3101, https://doi.org/10.1158/0008-5472.SABCS-09-3101; R. Jerath, M. W. Crawford, V. A. Barnes, et al., "Self-Regulation of Breathing as a Primary Treatment for Anxiety," *Applied Psychophysiology and Biofeedback* 40 (April 2015): 107–15, https://doi.org/10.1007/s10484-015-9279-8; and H. Cramer, R. Lauche, A. Paul, and G. Dobos, "Mindfulness-Based Stress Reduction for Breast Cancer—A Systematic Review and Meta-Analysis," *Current Oncology* 19, no. 5 (2012): 343–52, https://doi.org/10.3747/co.19.1016.
2. C. N. Joseph, C. Porta, G. Casucci, N. Casiraghi, M. Maffeis, M. Rossi, et al., "Slow Breathing Improves Arterial Baroreflex Sensitivity and Decreases Blood Pressure in Essential Hypertension," *Hypertension* 46, no. 4 (2005): 714–18, https://doi.org/10.1161/01.HYP.0000179581.68566.7d.

CHAPTER 6: BE YOUR OWN ADVOCATE

1. American Cancer Society, "Hormone Therapy for Breast Cancer," last revised September 28, 2025, https://www.cancer.org/cancer/types/breast-cancer/treatment/hormone-therapy-for-breast-cancer.html.

CHAPTER 7: REQUEST THE EXPERTISE OF PATIENT NAVIGATORS

1. M. Chen, V. S. Wu, D. Falk, C. Cheatham, J. Cullen, and R. Hoehn, "Patient Navigation in Cancer Treatment: A Systematic Review," *Current Oncology Reports* 26 (April 2024): 504–37, https://doi.org/10.1007/s11912-024-01514-9.

CHAPTER 11: FIND OUT IF A CLINICAL TRIAL IS RIGHT FOR YOU

1. Information adapted from reputable sources, including ClinicalTrials.gov, the National Institutes of Health (NIH), the National Cancer Institute (NCI), the World Health Organization (WHO), patient advocacy groups, and standard informed consent guidelines. This synthesis reflects established protocols and best practices for participating in clinical trials.
2. J. M. Unger, D. L. Hershman, C. Till, L. M. Minasian, R. U. Osarogiagbon, M. E. Fleury, et al., "When Offered to Participate: A Systematic Review and Meta-Analysis of Patient Agreement to Participate in Cancer Clinical Trials," *Journal of the National Cancer Institute* 113, no. 3 (2021): 244–57, https://doi.org/10.1093/jnci/djaa155.

CHAPTER 15: ORGANIZE MEDICAL BILLS AND INSURANCE DOCUMENTS

1. K. Thiboldeaux, *Your Cancer Road Map* (BenBella Books, 2021), 62.

CHAPTER 16: HOW NUTRITION CAN HELP YOU HEAL

1. A. M. Ryan, D. G. Power, L. Daly, S. J. Cushen, Ē. Ní Bhuachalla, and C. M. Prado, "Cancer-Associated Malnutrition, Cachexia and Sarcopenia: The Skeleton in the Hospital Closet 40 Years Later," *Proceedings of the Nutrition Society* 75, no. 2 (2016): 199–211, https://doi.org/10.1017/S002966511500419X.
2. Ryan et al., "Cancer-Associated Malnutrition, Cachexia and Sarcopenia."
3. Ryan et al., "Cancer-Associated Malnutrition, Cachexia and Sarcopenia."
4. M. Muscaritoli, S. Lucia, A. Farcomeni, V. Lorusso, V. Saracino, C. Barone, et al., "Prevalence of Malnutrition in Patients at First Medical Oncology Visit: The PreMiO Study," *Oncotarget* 8, no. 45 (2017): 79884–96, https://doi.org/10.18632/oncotarget.20168.

CHAPTER 17: WHERE TO FIND EMOTIONAL SUPPORT

1. J. Holt-Lunstad, T. B. Smith, and J. B. Layton, "Social Relationships and Mortality Risk: A Meta-Analytic Review," *PLoS Medicine* 7, no. 7 (2010): e1000316, https://doi.org/10.1371/journal.pmed.1000316.
2. M. Pinquart and P. R. Duberstein, "Associations of Social Networks with Cancer Mortality: A Meta-Analysis," *Critical Reviews in Oncology/Hematology* 75, no. 2 (2010): 122–37, https://doi.org/10.1016/j.critrevonc.2009.06.003; and J. M. Beasley, P. A. Newcomb, A. Trentham-Dietz, J. M. Hampton, R. M. Ceballos, L. Titus-Ernstoff, et al., "Social Networks and Survival After Breast Cancer Diagnosis," *Journal of Cancer Survivorship* 4 (July 2010): 372–80, https://doi.org/10.1007/s11764-010-0139-5.
3. C. H. Kroenke, C. Quesenberry, M. L. Kwan, C. Sweeney, A. Castillo, and B. J. Caan, "Social Networks, Social Support, and Burden in Relationships, and Mortality After

Breast Cancer Diagnosis in the Life After Breast Cancer Epidemiology (LACE) Study," *Breast Cancer Research and Treatment* 137 (January 2013): 261–71, https://doi.org/10.1007/s10549-012-2253-8.

4. National Cancer Institute, "Cancer Support Groups," last revised July 26, 2024, https://www.cancer.gov/about-cancer/coping/adjusting-to-cancer/support-groups.

CHAPTER 18: HOW GRATITUDE CAN IMPROVE YOUR RECOVERY

1. R. A. Emmons and M. E. McCullough, "Counting Blessings Versus Burdens: An Experimental Investigation of Gratitude and Subjective Well-Being in Daily Life," *Journal of Personality and Social Psychology 84, no.* 2 (2003): 377–89, https://doi.org/10.1037/0022-3514.84.2.377; R. A. Emmons, *Thanks! How the New Science of Gratitude Can Make You Happier* (Houghton Mifflin Harcourt, 2007); and R. A. Emmons and R. Stern, "Gratitude as a Psychotherapeutic Intervention," *Journal of Clinical Psychology 69, no.* 8 (2013): 846–55, https://doi.org/10.1002/jclp.22020.
2. Emmons and McCullough, "Counting Blessings Versus Burdens"; and R. Zahn, J. Moll, M. Paiva, G. Garrido, F. Krueger, E. D. Huey, et al., "The Neural Basis of Human Social Values: Evidence from Functional MRI," *Cerebral Cortex* 19, no. 2 (2009): 276–83, https://doi.org/10.1093/cercor/bhn080.

CHAPTER 19: MEDITATION

1. L. E. Carlson, R. Doll, J. Stephen, P. Faris, R. Tamagawa, E. Drysdale, et al., "Randomized Controlled Trial of Mindfulness-Based Cancer Recovery Versus Supportive Expressive Group Therapy for Distressed Survivors of Breast Cancer," *Journal of Clinical Oncology* 31, no. 25 (2013): 3119–26, https://doi.org/10.1200/jco.2012.47.5210.
2. F. Zeidan and D. R. Vago, "Mindfulness Meditation-Based

Pain Relief: A Mechanistic Account," *Annals of the New York Academy of Sciences* 1373, no. 1 (2016): 114–27, https://doi.org/10.1111/nyas.13153.

3. R. J. Davidson, J. Kabat-Zinn, J. Schumacher, M. Rosenkranz, D. Muller, S. F. Santorelli, et al., "Alterations in Brain and Immune Function Produced by Mindfulness Meditation," *Psychosomatic Medicine 65,* no. 4 (2003): 564–70, https://doi.org/10.1097/01.PSY.0000077505.67574.E3.
4. M. Speca, L. E. Carlson, E. Goodey, and M. Angen, "A Randomized, Wait-List Controlled Clinical Trial: The Effect of a Mindfulness Meditation-Based Stress Reduction Program on Mood and Symptoms of Stress in Cancer Outpatients," *Psychosomatic Medicine 62,* no. 5 (2000): 613–22, https://doi.org/10.1097/00006842-200009000-00004.
5. E. Foley, A. Baillie, M. Huxter, M. Price, and E. Sinclair, "Mindfulness-Based Cognitive Therapy for Individuals Whose Lives Have Been Affected by Cancer: A Randomized Controlled Trial," *Journal of Consulting and Clinical Psychology* 78, no. 1 (2010): 72–79, https://doi.org/10.1037/a0017566; and B. L. Fredrickson, M. A. Cohn, K. A. Coffey, J. Pek, and S. M. Finkel, "Open Hearts Build Lives: Positive Emotions, Induced Through Loving-Kindness Meditation, Build Consequential Personal Resources," *Journal of Personality and Social Psychology 95,* no. 5 (2008): 1045–62, https://doi.org/10.1037/a0013262.
6. L. E. Carlson, M. Speca, K. D. Patel, and E. Goodey, "Mindfulness-Based Stress Reduction in Relation to Quality of Life, Mood, Symptoms of Stress, and Immune Parameters in Breast and Prostate Cancer Outpatients," *Psychosomatic Medicine 65, no.* 4 (2003): 571–81, https://doi.org/10.1097/01.psy.0000074003.35911.41; and Foley et al., "Mindfulness-Based Cognitive Therapy."
7. Leading cancer treatment centers, such as Memorial Sloan Kettering Cancer Center, MD Anderson Cancer Center,

and Mayo Clinic, have incorporated meditation and mindfulness programs into their patient care offerings. These programs are designed to complement conventional cancer treatments by addressing the psychological and emotional needs of patients. Additionally, the World Health Organization (WHO) and other international health bodies have acknowledged the importance of psychosocial support, including mindfulness and meditation, in cancer care.

CHAPTER 20: GUIDED IMAGERY

1. M. L. Rossman, *Guided Imagery for Self-Healing* (H. J. Kramer, 2000).
2. D. Tusek, J. M. Church, and V. W. Fazio, "Guided Imagery as a Coping Strategy for Perioperative Patients," *AORN Journal* 66, no. 4 (1997): 644–49, https://doi.org/10.1016/s0001-2092(06)62917-7; J. Gubili, S. Corcoran, and T. Bao, "What the Evidence Says About Guided Imagery in Oncologic Care," *ONS Voice*, January 18, 2021, https://voice.ons.org/news-and-views/01-2021/what-the-evidence-says-about-guided-imagery-in-oncologic-care; A. Charalambous, M. Giannakopoulou, E. Bozas, Y. Marcou, P. Kitsios, and L. Paikousis, "Guided Imagery and Progressive Muscle Relaxation as a Cluster of Symptoms Management Intervention in Patients Receiving Chemotherapy: A Randomized Control Trial," *PLoS One* 11, no. 6 (2016): e0156911, https://doi.org/10.1371/journal.pone.0156911; G. De Paolis, A. Naccarato, F. Cibelli, A. D'Alete, C. Mastroianni, L. Surdo, et al., "The Effectiveness of Progressive Muscle Relaxation and Interactive Guided Imagery as a Pain-Reducing Intervention in Advanced Cancer Patients: A Multicentre Randomised Controlled Non-Pharmacological Trial," *Complementary Therapies in Clinical Practice* 34 (February 2019): 280–87, https://doi.org/10.1016/j.ctcp.2018.12.014; and M. J.

Mahdizadeh, B. Tirgari, O. S. R. R. Abadi, and K. Bahaadinbeigy, "Guided Imagery: Reducing Anxiety, Depression, and Selected Side Effects Associated with Chemotherapy," *Clinical Journal of Oncology Nursing* 23, no. 5 (2019): E87–E92, https://doi.org/10.1188/19.CJON.E87-E92.

3. Mahdizadeh et. al., "Guided Imagery"; Tusek et al., "Guided Imagery."
4. M. Weber, "Guided Imagery Reduces Stress and Anxiety in Patients Undergoing Radiation Therapy," *CURE*, December 11, 2009, www.curetoday.com/view/guided-imagery-reduces-stress-and-anxiety-in-patients-undergoing-radiation-therapy.
5. Rogel Cancer Center, "Finding Calm Within," *Thrive*, Spring 2007, University of Michigan Health, www.rogelcancercenter.org/living-with-cancer/mind-body-and-side-effects/finding-calm-within.
6. De Paolis et al., "Guided Imagery as a Pain-Reducing Intervention."
7. B. L. Gruber, N. R. Hall, S. P. Hersh, and P. Dubois, "Immune System and Psychological Changes in Metastatic Cancer Patients Using Relaxation and Guided Imagery: A Pilot Study," *Scandinavian Journal of Behaviour Therapy* 17, no. 1 (1988): 25–46, https://doi.org/10.1080/16506078809455814.
8. Mahdizadeh et al., "Guided Imagery."
9. S. Karagozoglu, F. Tekyasar, and F. A. Yilmaz, "Effects of Music Therapy and Guided Visual Imagery on Chemotherapy-Induced Anxiety and Nausea-Vomiting," *Journal of Clinical Nursing* 22, no. (1-2) (2013): 39–50, https://doi.org/10.1111/jocn.12030.
10. J. Brajtbord, A. Dhruva, S. Reddy, and S. Porten, "Study Examines Guided Imagery Meditation for Cancer Surgery Patients," UCSF Department of Urology, February 24, 2016, https://urology.ucsf.edu/news/all/201602/study-examines-guided-imagery-meditation-cancer-surgery-patients; and

C. Álvarez-García and Z. Ş Yaban, "The Effects of Preoperative Guided Imagery Interventions on Preoperative Anxiety and Postoperative Pain: A Meta-Analysis," *Complement Therapies in Clinical Practice* 38 (February 2020):101077, https://doi.org/10.1016/j.ctcp.2019.101077.

11. Charalambous et al., "Guided Imagery and Progressive Muscle Relaxation."

CHAPTER 23: QIGONG

1. K. S. Cohen, *The Way of Qigong: The Art and Science of Chinese Energy Healing* (Ballantine Books, 1997).

CHAPTER 24: FELDENKRAIS

1. N. Doidge, *The Brain's Way of Healing: Remarkable Discoveries and Recoveries from the Frontiers of Neuroplasticity* (Viking, 2015).

CHAPTER 25: REIKI

1. K. L. Tsang, L. E. Carlson, and K. Olson, "Pilot Crossover Trial of Reiki Versus Rest for Treating Cancer-Related Fatigue," *Integrative Cancer Therapies* 6 no. 1 (2007): 25–35, https://doi.org/10.1177/1534735406298986; X. Guo, Y. Long, Z. Qin, and Y. Fan, "Therapeutic Effects of Reiki on Interventions for Anxiety: A Meta-Analysis," *BMC Palliative Care* 23, no. 147 (2024), https://doi.org/10.1186/s12904-024-01439-x; S. Zadro and P. Stapleton, "Does Reiki Benefit Mental Health Symptoms Above Placebo?," *Frontiers in Psychology* 13 (July 2022): 897312, https://doi.org/10.3389/fpsyg.2022.897312; L. Fayed, "The Benefits of Reiki Therapy During Cancer Treatment," Verywell Health, last modified February 24, 2023, www.verywellhealth.com/reiki-therapy-513540; K. Olson, J. Hanson, and M. Michaud, "A Phase II Trial of Reiki for the Management of Pain in Advanced

Cancer Patients," *Journal of Pain and Symptom Management* 26, no. 5 (2003): 990–97, https://doi.org/10.1016/s0885-3924(03)00334-8; and C. M. Seluzicki, S. Corcoran, and J. J. Mao, "What Does the Evidence Say About Reiki for Cancer?," ONS Voice, November 21, 2019, www.ons.org/publications-research/voice/news-views/11-2019/what-does-evidence-say-about-reiki-cancer.

FINANCIAL RESOURCES:

1. Centers for Disease Control and Prevention, "Fast Facts: Health and Economic Costs of Chronic Conditions," July 12, 2024, www.cdc.gov/chronic-disease/data-research/facts-stats/index.html; and Centers for Disease Control and Prevention, "Heart Disease Facts," October 24, 2024, www.cdc.gov/heart-disease/data-research/facts-stats/index.html.
2. C. E. Fasola, "The Cost of Cancer," *SERO* (blog), February 23, 2025, accessed March 20, 2025, https://treatcancer.com/blog/cost-of-cancer.
3. T. G. Knight, M. Aguiar, M. Robinson, A. Martin, T. Chen, R. Bose, et al., "Financial Toxicity Intervention Decreases Mortality in High Risk Hematologic Malignancy Patients," *Blood* 136, no. s1 (2020): 14–15, https://doi.org/10.1182/blood-2020-137222.

About the Author

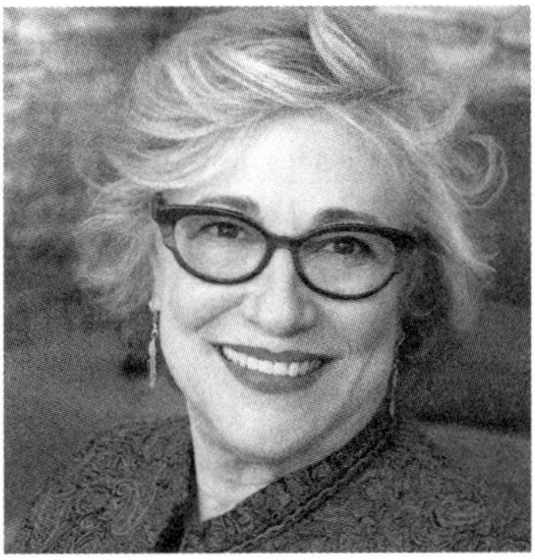

When journalist Jennifer Omholt was diagnosed with stage 3 breast cancer, her son was just 16 months old. Overwhelmed by the trauma of her diagnosis and the flood of medical information, she searched for a practical guide to help her navigate the weeks and months ahead. Yet no such guide existed. So she set out to create the resource she wished she'd had. *Just Diagnosed* draws on her resilience as a long-term survivor, blending personal insight, medical expertise, and evidence-based integrative strategies. She lives in the San Francisco Bay Area with her husband and their Maine Coon cat, Aristaeus, and is dedicated to helping newly diagnosed patients find clarity and strength in the critical first weeks after diagnosis.

To learn more, visit www.justdiagnosed.com.

Author photo courtesy of the author